Sound Clash

Jamaican Dancehall Culture at Large

Carolyn Cooper

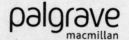

First published 2004 by
PALGRAVE MACMILLAN™
175 Fifth Avenue, New York, N.Y. 10010 and
Houndmills, Basingstoke, Hampshire, England RG21 6XS.
Companies and representatives throughout the world.

PALGRAVE MACMILLAN IS THE GLOBAL ACADEMIC IMPRINT OF THE PAL-GRAVE MACMILLAN

division of St. Martin's Press, LLC and of Palgrave Macmillan Ltd. Macmillan® is a registered trademark in the United States, United Kingdom and other countries. Palgrave is a registered trademark in the European Union and other countries.

ISBN 1-4039-6425-4 hardback
ISBN 1-4039-6424-6 paperback

Library of Congress Cataloging-in-Publication Data
Cooper, Carolyn, 1950–
    Sound clash : Jamaican dancehall culture at large / Carolyn Cooper.
        p. cm.
    Includes bibliographical references and index.
    ISBN 1-4039-6425-4 (cl) / 1-4039-6424-6 (pbk.)
     1. Jamaica—Social life and customs. 2. Music and dance—Jamaica—History. 3. Popular music—Jamaica—History and criticism. 4. Dance halls—Social aspects—Jamaica. 5. Women dancers—Sexual behavior—Jamaica. 6. Ragga (Music) 7. Popular culture—Jamaica. I. Title.

F1874.C663 2004
306.4'846'097292—dc22

                                                                           2003060161

A catalogue record for this book is available from the British Library.

Design by planettheo.com

First edition: September 2004
D 10 9 8 7 6 5 4 3 2

Printed in the United States of America.

Contents

Acknowledgments

My first debt of gratitude is to those of my colleagues at the University of the West Indies who have variously endorsed and contested my efforts to locate Jamaican dancehall culture firmly within the academy. Endorsement confirms value; contestation sharpens wits. I am particularly grateful to Joseph Pereira, deputy principal, director of the Institute of Caribbean Studies, and former dean of the Faculty of Humanities and Education on the Mona campus, with whom I first shared the idea of establishing at the university a center for research and teaching on reggae. His enthusiastic response provided the impetus to begin the prolonged institutionalization process. I am equally grateful to Hubert Devonish, my second convert, whose support for the project was manifested in immediate action. With evangelical zeal he quickly wrote the first draft of the project document that delineated the rationale and scope of the proposed center as a multidisciplinary enterprise.

Hubert, who is professor of Caribbean linguistics at Mona, has been a dependable ally not only in traversing the minefield of university politics but also in helping me refine my argument as the book developed. He has functioned as an often-cantankerous copilot on my many flights of fancy. It was Hubert who observed that my provocative representation of female sexuality in the dancehall as an emancipatory body politics was, indeed, an acknowledgment of the survival and adaptation of African female fertility rituals in the diaspora. This distillation of the essence of my argument gave a new respectability to my transgressive reading of the eroticized black female body in contemporary Jamaican dancehall culture, which other colleagues had simply dismissed as politically incorrect, if not downright misogynist.

I am also indebted to Hubert for permitting me to reproduce here our joint paper, "A Tale of Two States: Language, Lit/orature and the Two Jamaicas"; which, as chapter 10, has been somewhat revised and given a new title more appropriate to its present context: "The Dancehall Transnation: Language, Lit/orature, and Global Jamaica."[1] Collaborative writing tests the limits of friendship. In this case, writing across disciplines aggravated the process. Linguistics is an exact science, as Hubert would have it. Happily, literary/cultural studies is not, despite the scientific pretensions of the ubiquitous Greco-Latin neologisms. Nevertheless, Hubert and I managed to negotiate across disciplinary boundaries, and we are both quite satisfied with the outcome of the experiment.

I especially appreciate the sustained support of Cecil Gutzmore, lecturer in Carribean Studies at Mona and coauthor of chapter 1, "Border Clash: Sites of Contestation." I must thank him for access to his magnificent library and his extensive collection of dancehall CDs that made it so very easy for me to research the song texts I document here. Cecil has been a sounding board for many of the ideas I elaborate here. In particular, he readily responded to my request that he read the first draft of the paper on the politics of location that I was preparing for a 1998 symposium entitled "Partitions/Borders/Statism" at Trinity College, Hartford. Gutzmore's critique was so incisive—defining other sites of contestation than I had initially demarcated; and generously writing them into the text in expansive detail—that it seemed only fair to acknowledge his input as coauthorship. His insights substantially reconfigured the terrain of that draft paper.

I am also indebted to Romae Gordon, then a student at Trinity College, who insisted that I attend that important Hartford symposium and persuaded her teachers to invite me. Romae felt it imperative to include a Jamaican perspective in the deliberations. Indeed, I must acknowledge the input of the various audiences who have responded so thoughtfully to presentations of these papers at academic conferences. Their helpful comments have sharpened my argument. The international conference on African Diaspora Studies, convened in 1998 at the University of California, Berkeley, by Percy Hintzen, then director of the African American Studies Center, was an excellent occasion on which to present an expanded version of the Trinity College conference paper. At that important panafricanist conference I met many colleagues who continue to affirm the integrity of the borderline guerrilla scholarship in which I am engaged.

Outstanding among them is the Nigerian sociologist Oyeronke Oyewumi, whose iconoclastic book, *The Invention of Women: Making an African Sense of Western Gender Discourses,* like the online *jendajournal* she coedits, rereads globalizing western feminist discourses on gender through the lens of *jenda*—culture-specific African/diasporic ideology and *livity,* to use a Rastafari neologism, meaning way of life. That apparently idiosyncratic spelling "jenda" does represent accurately the way in which many global African speakers pronounce the colonized English word "gender." The phonetic spelling thus signals particularity of meaning and the localized politics of representation, issues that preoccupy me in my work on Jamaican popular culture. Ronke was instrumental in arranging for me to visit the University of California, Santa Barbara, where I presented in 2001 the paper "'Mama, Is That You?': Erotic Disguise in the Films *Dancehall Queen* and *Babymother.*"

That paper, reproduced here as chapter 4, has been much presented. I am committed to the ecological principle of recycling and firmly believe that no good academic paper should be performed only once. Each audience hears/reads the text differently and provides new contexts for its elaboration. I must acknowledge the graciousness of Professor Kofi Anyidoho and Dr. Aloysius Denkabe of the University of Ghana, Legon, who welcomed my offer to present the paper there in 2000, where it resonated with a wide range of scholars in literature and theater arts. Both films were screened and generated a lively cross-cultural dialogue about the representation of the black female body in public discourses in Africa and the diaspora.

I must thank Charmaine Warren, dance scholar and a demanding teacher—I took classes with her one summer at the College of the Visual and Performing Arts in Jamaica—for introducing my work on Jamaican popular culture to Sally Sommers, formerly of Duke University and now professor of dance at Florida State University, Tallahassee. Sally invited me to participate in the July 2000 international conference, "Dancing in the Millennium," which brought together practitioners and theorists on dance from a wide range of academic institutions and dance organisations. At that conference I presented an early version of chapter 3, "Lady Saw Cuts Loose: Female Fertility Rituals in the Dancehall," on a panel that examined club dancing. This border crossing into dance scholarship was a most illuminating experience. Coming from literary studies and feeling embattled in my attempts to take dancehall culture seriously, I was gratified to meet other scholars similarly engaged in researching the popular. Further, many of the familiar "postcolonial" issues surrounding the representation of the body, for example, manifest themselves most acutely in the corpus of dance theory and practice. I was subsequently invited to deliver the keynote address at the 2001 Dance Conference of the University of California Graduate Students, convened at the Davis campus.

I particularly value the local Jamaican/Caribbean audiences who, over the last decade, have responded so passionately to the readings of dancehall culture I have offered at academic conferences and, more widely, in the electronic and print media. I must acknowledge the following broadcasting houses in Jamaica and elsewhere for having amplified my voice: the morning radio talk show *The Breakfast Club,* hosted by Beverley Anderson-Manley and Anthony Abrahams; Television Jamaica's *Entertainment Report,* hosted by Anthony Miller; *Perspective* and *Man and Woman Story*—the latter program I cohosted with psychologist and self-styled "change agent" Leachim Semaj; CVM Television's *Question Time* and *Impact;* KLAS FM's *My Place;* FAME FM's *Uncensored* and Mutabaruka's *Cutting Edge* program on IRIE FM; the Caribbean Broadcasting Union's *Talk Caribbean Television* program; various BBC, Channel Four, and Black Audio Collective programs on Caribbean culture; Germany's new up-market reggae/dancehall magazine, *Riddim,* published by the Munich-based Piranha Media, with a circulation of 40,000. These media houses have afforded me numerous opportunities to participate in public debate on a host of contentious social issues such as language politics, gender, and, especially, Jamaican dancehall culture.

My weekly newspaper column written for the *Jamaica Observer* between 1993 and 1998 provided a valuable medium for me to test at the popular level a number of the "academic" issues that I explore here. In its very naming, "(W)uman Tong(ue)," the column signaled bilingualism and thus contested the myth of a monolingual Jamaican national identity articulated exclusively in English. This issue is fully addressed in chapter 10. All those hostile letters to the editor, attacking me for using the Jamaican language on the editorial page of a national newspaper and for making "controversial" statements about Jamaican popular culture, do have their important place. Indeed, my detractors, even more so than my sympathizers, have compelled me to pay close attention to the details of my argument for which I am most grateful.

I gratefully acknowledge the Gleaner company for permission to reproduce photographs and edited captions from its archives and I especially thank Ms. Sheree Rhoden, research assistant, for her painstaking work to identify appropriate images.

For Louise Frazer-Bennett, 1953-2003, founding president of the
Sound System Association of Jamaica;
and for the dancehall massive—a yard and abroad.

Word, Sound, and Power

Dem sound deh a no threat
Dem sound as if me deh a yard
A listen mi cassette[1]

—Cocoa Tea

. . . globalization must never be read as a simple process of cultural homogenization; it is always an articulation of the local, of the specific and the global. Therefore, there will always be specificities—of voices, of positioning, of identity, of cultural traditions, of histories, and these are the conditions of enunciation which enable us to speak.[2]

—Stuart Hall

Cultural Studies in the age of globalization is embedded in a network of transnational discourses that appear to privilege the cosmopolitan and devalue the currency of the local. Indeed, the culture-specific nature of these "global" discourses is not readily conceded. Globalization, that cunning euphemism for the old imperial politics of appropriation and exploitation, resonates differently across the globe even as an economic system. Globalization as an ideology of cultural homogenization is especially problematic for those peoples of the world who are collectively constituted as the ever-marginalized consumers of the waste products of metropolitan societies—whether outdated manufactured commodities, stale food, or cultural theories that have long outlived their sell-by date.[3] Ubiquitous postmodernist conceptions of the self as a hybridized mass of displaced, free-floating, multiple signifiers are quite irrelevant in supposedly "postcolonial" societies where hardworking people struggle to articulate a coherent sense of identity in resistance to the destabilizing imperative of neocolonial social, economic, and political forces.

This study of Jamaican dancehall culture is stubbornly rooted in a politics of place that claims a privileged space for the local and asserts the authority of the native as speaking subject. However, the local is decidedly not conceived as a narrowly insular, uniformly flat landscape, cut off from currents of thought beyond its shores. Indeed, an island is a frontier. Seemingly bounded on all sides by the sea, it does have porous borders and remains open to multiple influences. The sea, after all, is not a constricting dam, but a vast waterway across which Caribbean peoples and our cultures constantly recirculate to continents of origin and beyond.

This collection of essays, leisurely written over the last decade or so, is an elaboration of my exploratory 1990 essay, published in *Jamaica Journal*, "Slackness Hiding from Culture: Erotic Play in the Dancehall," the first academic study of Jamaican dancehall culture, as far as I can tell.[4] Encoding subversion, the title of that essay, taken from a composition by DJ Josey Wales, celebrates the cunning wiles of slackness; the subtitle, foregrounding the erotic, underscores the ambiguities of disgust and desire in the dancehall imaginary: feminized, seductive slackness simultaneously resisting and enticing respectable culture.[5] In Jamaican usage, the English word "slackness" has almost exclusively sexual overtones and is synonymous with licentiousness—"libertine, lascivious, lewd" behavior— to cite the alliterative *Oxford English Dictionary (OED)* definition of the word. But the license in the English licentiousness is often repressed in its Jamaican equivalent and only the censure remains.

The *Dictionary of Jamaican English* does not have an entry on "slackness." But it does define a "slack" as "1. a slovenly person. 2. a woman of loose morals." The gender bias is evident in this unsettling shift of meaning from the domain of the literal and superficial—dress/appearance—to that of the metaphorical and substantive—moral conduct. The gender-neutral "slovenly person" becomes the gender-specific "woman of loose morals." Modes of un/dress have long been read as signs of the moral condition of both men and women, as far back as the Garden of Eden. Thus, for example, the delightful *OED* citation, dated 1700: "Marriage . . . often melts down a Beau into an errant sloven." Here the sloven errantry of the dissolute Beau seems to be both sartorial and moral. But in the Jamaican context, slackness becomes essentialized as the generic condition of immoral woman, not man. Women are supposed to be the perennial guardians of private and public morality; men are allowed to extemporize.

In that pioneering essay, I analyze the lyrics of representative DJs and identify five major thematic groupings of song texts: (1) songs that celebrate DJing itself; (2) dance songs that vigorously invite participants to "shock out" and party; (3) songs of social commentary on a variety of issues, for example, ghetto violence and hunger; (4) songs that focus on sexual/gender relations—by far the largest number in the sample; and (5) songs that explicitly speak to the slackness/culture opposition. On the basis of a detailed content analysis of approximately fifty song texts, I conclude that the dancehall constitutes a discrete, if evidently not discreet, culture; it is a dedicated space for the flamboyant performing of sexuality. And I identify subversion as a quintessential feature of the promiscuous culture of the dancehall. I here deploy "promiscuous" in the original, asexual Latinate sense of the word—"mixed together."

I argue that slackness, though often conceived and critiqued as an exclusively sexual and *politically* conservative discourse, can be much more permissively theorized as a radical, underground confrontation with the patriarchal gender ideology and the duplicitous morality of fundamentalist Jamaican society. Slackness is not mere sexual looseness, though it certainly is that. Slackness is a contestation of conventional definitions of law and order; an undermining of consensual standards of decency. At large, slackness is the antithesis of restrictive uppercase Culture. It thus challenges the rigid status quo of social exclusivity and one-sided moral authority valorized by the Jamaican elite. Slackness demarcates a space for alternative definitions of "culture."

My academic engagement with Jamaican dancehall culture thus began from the disciplinary perspective of literary studies with the careful reading of DJ lyrics. Critical attention to verbal meaning does not, of course, preclude sensitivity to the total context of production and performance of these lyrical texts. My 1989-1990 essay became the penultimate chapter of a book, *Noises in the Blood: Orality, Gender and the "Vulgar" Body of Jamaican Popular Culture,* that located marginalized popular culture texts within their particular sociopolitical and aesthetic context.[6] I conclude that study of Jamaican popular culture in this way: "In attempting to retheorise marginality and power, these essays begin with primary texts, centring the ideological narrative on close readings of the texts themselves. This repositioning of the displaced 'primary' text at the centre of the theorising project is itself a subversive act. Instead of imposing polysyllabic, imported theories of cultural production on these localised Jamaican texts, I have attempted to discover what the texts themselves can be made to tell us about the nature of cultural production in our centres of learning."[7]

I was engaged in a cultural studies project that was very much in tune with work that was taking place elsewhere. In the words of cultural theorists Cary Nelson, Paula Treichler, and Lawrence Grossberg: "Cultural studies does not require us to repudiate elite cultural forms—or simply to acknowledge . . . that distinctions between elite and popular cultural forms are themselves the products of relations of power. Rather, cultural studies requires us to identify the operation of specific practices, of how they continuously reinscribe the line between legitimate and popular culture, and of what they accomplish in specific contexts. At the same time, cultural studies must constantly interrogate its own connection to contemporary relations of power, its own stakes."[8]

Given my scrupulous attention to the wider social and political meanings of cultural texts and my constant questioning of my own placement in the academy as a scholar engaged in "borderline" research on the popular, I must problematize the rather ponderous critique of my work on dancehall culture offered by Norman Stolzoff in his 2000 book on Jamaican sound systems:

> What is wrong with many analyses of dancehall culture is the way that they either start at the level of the analysis of cultural texts (song lyrics), or they go straight to an aesthetic or ethical critique of the work without examining the way that the text is produced or consumed and what effects these processes have on the text. Studies such as Cooper's (1993) miss the way that dancehall is integrated into daily life and how the meanings of songs are contingent on historical, productive, and performative factors. Additionally, these overly hermeneutic interpretations miss other forms of performance, such as dance and other bodily practices, which cannot be easily read as symbolic text. For example, vocal and musical quality are as important to listeners as is the strictly lexical register.[9]

Stolzoff's bumptious generalizations, apparently intended to valorize his presumably all-encompassing anthropological approach to Jamaican dancehall culture, misrepresent the range and resonance of my work. I make it quite clear in the introductory chapter of *Noises in the Blood* that I am very much aware of how much the "meanings of songs are contingent on historical, productive, and performative factors" and how important are "forms of performance, such as dance and other bodily practices"— though I choose, nevertheless, to privilege the analysis of lyrics, for good reason: Pleasure in the word is a fundamental element of the total theater of the dancehall. Indeed, language, in the most literal sense of the word, is the primary medium through which the DJs articulate their preoccupations and communicate directly with their receptive audiences. Performance is dialogue with an audience that speaks back in no uncertain terms.

Furthermore, in Jamaica, the language of the DJs is the most contested component of their total performance repertoire, and what they say is often dismissed as pure nonsense by elitist critics of the genre or, worse, is deemed seditious. The new policing of the DJs' use of "bad" words in their public performances is an extreme example of the society's perennial obsession with the language of the dancehall—both its rhetorical tropes as well as its unselfconscious affirmation of the devalued "patwa" mother tongue of the vast majority of Jamaicans. In 2003, middle-class DJ Sean Paul [Henriques] was served with a summons for his use of profanity during his performance at the annual reggae festival, Sumfest. Journalist Mark Cummings reports the DJ's account of his behavior as an act of protest in solidarity with working-class DJs who are routinely charged by the police: "'Artistes curse on the stage, I have done it before at a show in Negril in April and somebody pointed it out to me and said that: don't you think that it is unfair that others have cursed and got summons, and you curse and did not get any?' the deejay said. 'It's an 'unbalance' scale and because I have an international appeal and a voice right now, I am using it to highlight it.'"[10] Sean Paul's principled, militant position is undermined by the penitent headline of the report: "I have learnt my lesson—*Sean Paul.*"

Less equivocally, Anthony B's respectful line in the refractory song "Nah Vote Again"—"talk like Miss Lou, mi no talk like foreigner"[11] [I talk like Miss Lou, I don't talk like a foreigner]—acknowledges the DJ's affiliation to an indigenous performance tradition that is articulated in "nation language," to cite the work of the Barbadian griot, Kamau Brathwaite. Anthony B here pays respect to national icon, Miss Lou, the Honorable Dr. Louise Bennett-Coverley—poet, actress, folklorist, cultural ambassador—the most celebrated advocate of the reclamation of the Jamaican mother tongue from the condition of barbarism contemptuously assigned to the language and its habitual speakers.

In focusing on this "outlaw" language in my study of Jamaican dancehall culture, I was reclaiming the power of the indigenous voice and the nativist worldview of the marginalized wordsmiths, especially the DJs. As I argue in *Noises in the Blood:*

> The lyrics of the reggae musician and the DJ, related in performance terms to the poetry of Bennett, Breeze and Smith constitute the fourth group of texts to be examined. The least scribal of the texts under consideration, they become the most de-contextualised in the kind of close verbal/textual reading to which they are subjected here. The cautionary Brathwaite epigraph from *History of the Voice* draws deliberate attention to the sound and not simply the sight of the text. The basic limitation of this sighted focus on lyrics is that relatively little attention is given to the analysis of the non-verbal elements of production and performance: melody, rhythm, the body in dance and the dancefloor itself as a space of spectacle and display. Relatively little attention is paid to the institutions of music production or to assessing the degree to which modes of production and performance reinforce or undermine the power relations at play in the lyrics. But the value of the analysis of disembodied lyrics is that the "noise" of the reggae musician and DJ is heard as intelligible and worthy of serious critical attention.[12]

To be fair to Stolzoff, I must concede the possibility that perhaps he read only the chapter on dancehall culture, not the whole book. He did not hear all the noises. So he would have missed that expansive statement in which I define the parameters of the study. Nevertheless, had he read the dancehall chapter carefully enough, he would have noticed this compressed restatement of the earlier argument: "the DJ's verbal art originates in an inclusivist neo-African folk aesthetic—a carnivalesque fusion of word, music and movement around the centre pole, and on the common ground of the dance floor."[13]

In addition, Stolzoff does not appear to fully understand the significance of the point I make about the marginalized place of the DJ's lyrics in the scribal/oral literary continuum in Jamaica. In an extended footnote in his chapter on the career path of the DJ, Stolzoff observes that "it is important to note that while DJing is an oral form, as Carolyn Cooper stresses in *Noises in the Blood* (1994: 136), it is not 'the furthest extreme of the scribal/oral/ literary continuum in Jamaica,' as she asserts. Writing down lyrics, if only for the sake of remembering them, is part and parcel of getting involved and learning the DJ art form."[14] Stolzoff's formulation, "scribal/oral/literary continuum," is not an accurate quotation. The insertion of that virgule after oral may be a simple typographical error. But it does distort my meaning. I intend both "scribal" and "oral" to equally modify "literary," thus ascribing equivalent weight to both modes of discourse.

Like Stolzoff, Black British sociologist and DJ William "Lezlee Lyrix" Henry takes me to task for seeming to suggest that all DJs, except for Lovindeer, are nonliterate. In a rousing critique in his unpublished 1997 Bachelor of Arts dissertation. Henry argues that "[t]he Jamaican cultural critic Carolyn Cooper's book *Noises in the blood* (1993) was hailed as a 'pathbreaking enterprise' because it took several aspects of Jamaican 'word-culture' seriously, as she evaluated the role of language in Jamaican 'popular culture.' However, her analysis of dancehall falls victim to the Eurocentric view (which she is obviously challenging) of bestowing more credibility on supposed 'literary skill,' as opposed to 'oral skill.'"[15]

Citing an example of his own lyrics, Henry sets out to demonstrate the "pitfalls of using a formal 'education' as a yardstick to measure an Afri-centric cultural perspective."[16] He argues that his composition "exempli-fies how those who deem themselves to be oppressed, can transculturally express their opinions amongst others who largely share their socio-cultural perspective, within this autonomous space."[17] He waxes lyrical:

At school the teachers taught me things like how to use a Lathe, couldah ask them any question bout when man live innah cave, if me ask them bout when black man down innah slave, them blush, turn red, them answer used to scathe, I will give you an example of an answer they gave, bloody trouble maker, get out the class, until you learn to behave. It happen so much times some refused to teach me, wouldn't let me innah them class them send me to the library, that's when I decided to learn my history, and the words of these Men did enlighten me, Malcolm X, Martin Luther King and Marcus Garvey, so all black people I advise you strongly, learn about your culture so you know your history. (Lezlee Lyrix. Ghetto-tone Sound Syst [*sic*] 1983)[18]

But the fact that some DJs *do* write down lyrics—as I myself make quite clear, in particular reference to the atypical Lloyd Lovindeer—does not invalidate my argument that "[w]ith the DJs there is no presumption of an essentially 'scribal' literary tradition as the context of performance."[19] Indeed, I further argue in *Noises in the Blood* that "[t]he literariness of the DJ's art is thus subsumed in the totalising function of the dance. By contrast, the origins of the work of a neo-oral writer like Louise Bennett, whose poetry seems close in spirit to the pure orality of DJ performance, can be traced to both oral and scribal literary forms. Bennett's creolising of the inherited ballad form is, initially, an act of conscious literary modelling."[20] My primary point was *not* that all DJs are illiterate and therefore cannot write down their lyrics. Rather, I was locating the *performance tradition* of DJing within the broader scribal/oral literary continuum in Jamaica.

In 1989 (and, perhaps, even today) my recognition of the DJs' legitimate place on the literary continuum would have been seen by some skeptics as a clear sign of my suspension of critical judgment. Indeed, far from *dissing* "illiterate" DJs, as both Stolzoff and Henry appear to think that I am, I was instead reasserting the value of their resounding contribution to the corpus of literary production in Jamaica. I foreground Stolzoff's and, to a lesser degree, Henry's dismissal of my work in order to draw attention to a recurring "sound clash" in the academy between "local" and "foreign" scholars of Jamaican popular culture. The border-crossing DJ/academic "Lezlee Lyrix"/William Henry, born in the United Kingdom of Jamaican parents, clearly disrupts neat categories. His "outsiderness" is relative. Nevertheless, Henry does not seem to fully apprehend the cultural politics on the ground *a yard*—as distinct from in the United Kingdom. The marginalization of dancehall culture in elitist discourses in Jamaica is undeniable, more so almost a decade and a half ago.

I do understand Henry's dismay at my "confession" in *Noises in the Blood* that it was "[a]fter enforced hearing of these [DJ] songs over several months [that] I decided to give the lyrics more serious attention."[21] Indeed, my early inattentive dismissal of the lyrics of the DJs was, essentially, an ageist refusal to listen closely to the meaning of the sounds of youth culture. But in his enthusiasm to reprimand me for this error of judgment, Henry fails to acknowledge the obvious: My painstaking analysis of dancehall lyrics in *Noises in the Blood* is itself evidence of my recognition, however belated, of the value of that corpus of performance texts. Henry, writing in 1997, argues as if my sustained work on dancehall lyrics does not itself engender a critique of cultural marginalization in Jamaica. He pontificates:

> As I have demonstrated, for those people who are primarily working class Jamaicans, they are the margins. Therefore, any cultural forms associated with them will be not only marginal, but will reflect the marginalised world inhabited by those who appreciate the necessity and validity of these cultural forms. This outlook is evident in the following extract from a popular reggae/dancehall tune of 1997 by the Jamaican singer Everton Blender, as he explains; "It's a ghetto peoples song only them can sing this one, it's a song for the poor whose facing sufferation." Hence, any evaluation of these cultural forms should consider the fact that they represent the majority of not only the most historically disenfranchised and oppressed of all Jamaicans, but the majority of Jamaicans proper, which means they represent a marginalised majority. Therefore, I would wish to pose what is for me a most relevant question which is; how can anyone undertake to explore an "oral, popular word culture" and only *stumble* across one of the most relevant aspects of that "word culture," largely by mistake?[22]

Quite easily. The miracle is that I stumbled at all. Furthermore, I am routinely abused in the local media for that fall from academic and moral grace. A 2003 letter to the editor of the *Gleaner*, written by Iris Myrie, vice president of the Business and Professional Women's Club of Kingston, and which was given prominence as the "Letter of the Day," exemplifies my own marginalization on the periphery of conventional social respectability. My provocative reading of dancehall culture as a liberating space for African Jamaican women is sarcastically dismissed by Myrie who locates herself at a discreet distance from my supposedly "educated" position: "Some of us women at the lower end of the educational scale cannot understand how Dr. Cooper rationalises the concept of "uplifting people's self esteem" by constant bombardment and derogatory comments. The fact that many of these women dance to these songs, dress the part of men [?], compete with other women to attract their male cohorts, dress their young daughters to attract the males, is evidence that the conditioning has happened. To us some of the dancehall lyrics have been used to enslave, subjugate and demoralise women."[23]

Myrie employs a visceral image to convey her distaste at my argument, as she understands it: "The cathartic effect of the music spoken of by Dr. Cooper is like vomiting to relieve the stomach of over surfeit, but doing so on the street in view of everyone else, depositing it on people, spoiling everyone's appetite so as to ease your own discomfort. It is sickening! The fact that you are hurting gives you no right to sicken others."[24] This upstanding spokeswoman for the Business and Professional Women's Club, a foreigner in the world of the dancehall, does not appear even to entertain the possibility that the generic "everyone," on whose behalf she glibly dares to speak, might not share her presumption about what is appropriate public behavior—whether literal or metaphorical.

The problem of the relative authority of in/outsider perspectives is not limited to the domain of the popular or academia. Foreign experts of all kinds routinely tell us how best to understand and "develop" our society. The insider's perspective is constantly invalidated as the outsider positions him/herself as the "real" authority in these matters. My critique of the presumptuousness of some of these foreign experts should not itself be misinterpreted as evidence of a mere fit of pique, an attempt to jealously protect territorial borders from recolonizing invaders, armed this time round with laptops.

I certainly welcome all those non-Caribbean academics who do engage seriously with our culture, adding to the ample body of scholarship that we are consolidating locally and in the Caribbean diaspora. Indeed, Norman Stolzoff's comprehensive taxonomy of Jamaican sound systems is an excellent example of what can be achieved in this collaborative enterprise. He was formally attached to the African-Caribbean Institute of Jamaica as a research fellow during his period of fieldwork in Jamaica and received expert advice from professionals in the industry such as Louise Frazer-Bennett, founder and first president of the Sound System Association of Jamaica, who opened doors for him that might otherwise have remained closed. What I must contest is the hubris of some foreign experts who seem to deliberately set out to undermine local scholarship in order to aggrandize their own reputations. They thus provoke border clashes.

I first deploy the metaphor of the "border clash" in the 1995 Preface to the U.S. edition of *Noises in the Blood*, primarily to underscore a series of conflicts within Jamaican society around identity and the representation of the body politic. Issues of class, race, gender, sexuality, voice and language are central to this discourse. In dancehall culture, the "sound clash" between rival sound systems is often conceived as a "border clash"—a battle to guard one's position of superiority in the field from the encroachments of upstart "tin pan" sounds. For example, Sugar Minott's "Can't Cross the Border" illustrates the way in which an "out of order" sound boy can be forced to retreat after unsuccessfully trying to penetrate the impregnable barriers that are erected to defend territory.[25] Order must be maintained on the b/order. Indeed, the disorderly sound boy who foolishly attempts to challenge a top ranking sound system is quickly brought to order. Asserting his control of the border, Sugar Minott repeatedly declares, "a ya" [it's here].[26] The borderline is the precise intersection where he and his crew manifest their megawattage power. Sugar Minott polices the border with his clever play on words, exemplifying his own lyrical mastery of the conventions of the clash.

In the title of that preface, "Informing Cultural Studies: A Politics of Betrayal?" I interrogate the role of the cultural critic as informer, on the borderline, mediating between the disempowered "low" and the all-powerful "high," between "insider" and "outsider." In Jamaican dancehall culture the much-maligned "informer" occupies a morally ambiguous position. Giving information to authority figures such as the police is not a simple matter of good citizenship. Information is power that can be abused. So the informer is often perceived as a threat to his/her community, disclosing its vulnerabilities.

This perspective is evident, for example, in Tony Rebel's "Chatty Chatty," which opens with a disclaimer: "Well yu see, through [because] me no have notn fi [nothing to] hide/ All informer, step aside!"[27] The song is an indictment of "chatty chatty" informers who make life difficult for all those hustlers struggling to succeed by any means necessary. The characteristic Jamaican Creole reduplication, "chatty chatty," intensifies the repercussions of the informer's disclosures. The refrain, "A through yu chatty chatty mi can't live in peace/ Every lickle ting yu run gone fi police," turns on the ironic rhyme of "peace" and "police."[28] The presence of the police decreases the peace. Tony Rebel documents several instances in which a female informer carries tales to the police. The gender of the informer, who responds by denouncing the DJ as a liar, reinforces the stereotype of gossip as a feminized discourse. But the "carry go bring come" rhetoric of domesticated gossip assumes dangerous proportions when taken out of the domain of somewhat harmless rumor mongering; it can become the deadly game of giving information to ruthless law enforcement agents.

Selling "weed," for example, is still a criminal activity in Jamaica, though there have been several campaigns to change the laws that make even possession of marijuana for personal use a crime. Miss Chatty Chatty's nosiness jeopardizes the hustler's career prospects in this field:

> Mi a try a lickle [little] hustling a sell some weed
>
> Yu come [u]pon mi doorstep an yu find two herb seed
>
> Carry mi name gone a station to Sergeant Reid
>
> Through [because] yu a mi friend['s] baby-mother
>
> An mi know seh [that] yu a breed [are pregnant]
>
> Mi no waan do yu notn so yu fi tek heed
>
> [I don't want to hurt you so you better take heed]
>
> Leave people business and mek [let]dem succeed[29]

The element of threat in the denunciation of the informer is attenuated by the DJ's loyalty to the woman's partner, his friend; and because of his perception of her as a vulnerable pregnant woman. So she gets off with a verbal warning. Otherwise, she might have suffered grievous bodily harm.

The DJ turns to another illegal activity, bearing unlicensed firearms, and underscores the "normative" quality of this aspect of ghetto gun culture:

> Everybody done know how in di ghetto run
>
> Fi defend yuself yu ha fi have a little gun
>
> Di other night yu see me a brandish a magnum
>
> Yu gone a station an a labba yu mout [blab].[30]

This knowledge that "everybody" supposedly possesses can, in fact, become dangerous when it is isolated and used to implicate a particular individual, especially in the ghetto where trigger-happy policemen shoot first and ask questions later. They often do not need too much information in order to act. Indeed, a little knowledge can be a very dangerous thing: "An yu know how it go when dem ya policemen ya come/ A [it's] just buyaka, buyaka an a guy drop dong [down]."[31] The onomatopoeic "buyaka" is the sound of the barking gun.

Tony Rebel identifies yet another domain in which informing becomes a life-threatening activity—male/female relationships:

Pon mi father side mi have a lickle (younger) sister
Come check mi yeside (yesterday) from down a Manchester
Mi an her a reason, mi seh, pon a corner
Yu run gone a mi yard gone tell mi lover
When yu tell her weh [what] she look like an di description
She just seh, "A Rebel sister dat, man!"[32]

In this narrative of informing, the DJ's lover occupies the same position as the police—the authority figure to whom the chatty chatty woman relays provocative gossip. Fortunately for the DJ, in this instance, the putative "outside woman" turns out to be relative, about whom the lover is fully informed.

Tony Rebel, whose legal name is Patrick Barrett, is one of the older generation of DJs with a public image of impeccable respectability. In 2002 he was awarded the national honor, Order of Distinction (Officer Rank), for his contribution to music and entertainment. The program for the ceremony of investiture and presentation of national honors and awards notes that "[t]he honor of the Order may be conferred upon any citizen of Jamaica who renders outstanding and important services to Jamaica and upon any distinguished citizen of a country other than Jamaica. The motto of the Order is *Distinction through Service.*" That a DJ of such stature includes in his repertoire an attack on informers indicates the depth of public sentiment against this act of perceived betrayal. Admittedly, the DJ denounces the informer who discloses "every lickle thing." Presumably he would not object to informing on more weighty matters than selling weed and brandishing a Magnum.

The cultural critic as informer, precariously located in a danger zone at the crossroads, is as vulnerable to crossfire as any other informer. But, as I argue in that 1995 preface, the risks are worth the potential benefits—

the expected transfer of knowledge and empathy across communities of contrasting discourses and of apparently differing sensibilities. Successfully negotiated border crossings are the very essence of enlightened cultural studies. In the present study I document a series of forays I have made across the shifting borderline between "academic" and "popular" territory. I do not claim for this project the definitive authority of an encyclopedic study of Jamaican dancehall culture. I offer, instead, the specificity of my voice, positioning (*a ya*) and identity—to cite Stuart Hall and Cocoa Tea—as I try to make sense of the border clashes that characterize much of contemporary Jamaican society, and which are therefore often chronicled within the popular performance genres such as "roots" theater, dub poetry, and, especially, popular music.

Contemporary "rub a dub" Jamaican popular music, alternately labeled "dancehall," "ragga," and "dub" in its various contexts of production and performance, is much lamented both at home and abroad as a primal scream—a barbaric, degenerate, eschatological sound.[33] I suppose scatological as well. More broadly, Jamaican dancehall culture is commonly disparaged as a misogynist, homophobic, homicidal discourse that reduces both men and women to bare essentials: skeletal remains. In this dehumanizing caricature women are misrepresented as mindless bodies, (un)dressed and on display exclusively for male sexual pleasure. And men are stereotyped as dog-hearted predators stalking potential victims. It is the animal nature of both genders that is foregrounded. It is true that sex and violence—basic instincts—are recurring themes in the lyrics of both male and female DJs. Understandably so. The dancehall is, essentially, a heterosexual space (heterosexist, even) in which men and women play out eroticized gender roles in ritual dramas that can become violent.

But sex and violence, however primal, are not the only preoccupations of Jamaican dancehall culture. Powerful currents of explicitly political lyrics urgently articulate the struggle of the celebrants in the dance to reclaim their humanity in circumstances of grave economic hardship that force the animal out of its lair. Indeed, Jamaican dancehall culture celebrates the dance as a mode of theatrical self-disclosure in which the body speaks eloquently of its capacity to endure and transcend material deprivation. Furthermore, the politics of the dancehall is decidedly gendered: It is the body of the woman that is invested with absolute authority as men pay homage to the female principle.

Arguing transgressively for the freedom of women to claim a self-pleasuring sexual identity that may even be explicitly homoerotic, I propose that Jamaican dancehall culture at home and in the diaspora is best understood as a potentially liberating space in which working-class women and their more timid middle-class sisters assert the freedom to play out eroticized roles that may not ordinarily be available to them in the rigid social conventions of the everyday. The dancehall, thus conceived, is an erogenous zone in which the celebration of female sexuality and fertility is ritualized. In less subtle readings of the gender politics of the dancehall, this self-conscious female assertion of control over the representation of the body (and identity) is misunderstood and the therapeutic potential of the dancing body is repressed. Indeed, the joyous display of the female body in the dance is misperceived as a pornographic devaluation of woman.

In addition, the unapologetic materialism of dancehall culture, with its valorization of "bling bling"—all of the trappings of worldly success—is much derided by both self-appointed middle-class arbiters of "good" taste as well as by fundamentalist Christians who, in theory, mortify the flesh. But the desire to own an ornate gold chain, for example, is not essentially different from the pervasive middle-class Jamaican aspiration to acquire a house that could easily pass as a castle or the fundamentalist Christian's intention to walk on streets paved with gold. Indeed, Ian Boyne, Christian pastor and radio/television presenter in Jamaica, who ordinarily lashes out against dancehall culture, somewhat surprisingly attacks Christians as well for their materialism: "The Christianity which is really 'running things' in Jamaica today is the 'Bling-bling' Christianity. Through the widespread penetration of cable television and the existence of *Love TV*, Jamaicans are exposed to a brand of North American Christianity which is promoting a very jaundiced view of the gospel. It's called the health and wealth gospel and it teaches that prosperity is a divine right that is promised to every believer."[34] Boyne's self-righteousness aside, one must concede that the desire for gold—whether "sacred" or "secular"—originates in the common human desire to enjoy luxury. To cite Shakespeare's King Lear: "Allow not nature more than nature needs,/ Man's life is cheap as beast's."

In chapter 1, "Border Clash: Sites of Contestation," Cecil Gutzmore and I examine the unsettling politics of location in Jamaican dancehall culture. We identify and explore a wide range of conflicts—across performance genres and language barriers; between religious positions; across state borders; between ghetto youth and authority figures; across shifting lines of gender and sexual orientation; between the reggae generation and their ragamuffin children—that altogether illustrate the sophisticated way in which dancehall performers engage with Jamaican "roots, reality, and culture."

In chapter 2, "Slackness Personified: Representations of Female Sexuality in the Lyrics of Bob Marley and Shabba Ranks," I invoke Bob Marley, universal symbol of "conscious" reggae music at its finest, as the high point of reference against which to measure the failings/accomplishments of the contemporary generation of DJs. And I select Shabba Ranks as their lowly representative. I know that some purists would denounce the very yoking of the names Shabba Ranks and Bob Marley in the same sentence. Nevertheless, I think it imperative to listen carefully to what the DJs actually say and not to permit prejudice—in the literal sense of prejudgment—to determine our final evaluation of their work. Furthermore, I believe that we must rehumanize Bob Marley by taking him off the pedestal on which he has been firmly fixed and thus made inaccessible to the present generation of ghetto youth at ground level.

In an instructive interview with Anthony B, one of the most insightful of the new wave of Rastafari DJs, David Scott, editor of the incisive journal *Small Axe*, raises the matter of dis/respect for the language of the

DJs that manifests itself precisely as a refusal to pay attention to what they say:

> DS: Yu t[h]ink people—mi mean uptown people, di people who run di TV or radio station—don't have nuff [a lot of] respect fa [for] all like your music. Me no mean respect inna di sense dat dem mighta play di music (because dem mighta play di music an don't have no respect fi it) but inna di sense dat dem don't listen di vibe inna di music an to di lyrics weh inna it. Yu tink a so?[35]

Anthony B agrees with Scott and further raises the troubling issue of the homogenizing one-dimensionality of popular conceptions of what "culture music" ought to be; the DJ also contests the authority of Bob Marley as the singular voice of that genre:

> AB: Yeah, dat is di problem. Dem no spend time sidong [sitting down] an *listen* di sense inna it, man. Because why? Dem hook pon a type a music now dat to dem is di one culture-music dem a listen to. An is Bob Marley.[36]

To Scott's follow up question, "But why is that?" Anthony B gives an equally insightful response: "Bob Marley naa hurt them no more . . . [My music] an Bob Marley music. Is di same music, is just dat Bob Marley can't hurt them no more. Bob Marley can't say nothing new. Bob Marley can't see wa a go on [what's going on] now an seh [say] wa im woulda like fi seh. But I am here now, who can seh it."[37] Not only does Anthony B here acknowledge the continuities between his visionary message and that of Bob Marley but, somewhat heretically, he claims the power to speak on behalf of iconic Bob Marley, who has been silenced not only by physical death but much more insidiously, and ironically, by his apotheosis. Imprisoned in divinity, Bob Marley can no longer speak directly to the youth. So Rastafari DJs like Anthony B must chant their own version of his cultural message, riding the new youthful *riddims* [rhythms] of resistance against the system.

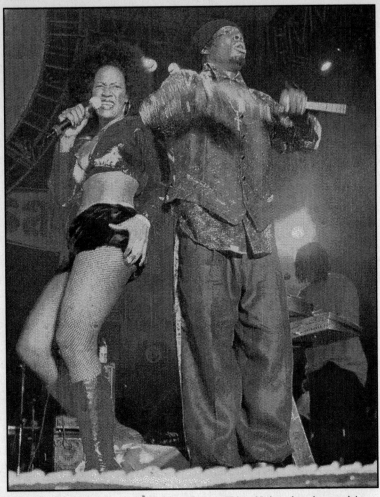

Shabba Ranks, Jamaica's first dancehall Reggae Grammy Kid, and Italee, talented poet and singer, as they performed at Sashi in August 2001 in Ocho Rios. Photo: Dennis Coke.

But even the tarnished "slackness" DJs like Shabba Ranks can shine in the reflected glory of Bob Marley. I examine the gender politics in the lyrics of both artists precisely because I wish to illustrate the ways in which contemporary dancehall culture is much more sophisticated than is usually assumed. Shabba Ranks, who is stereotypically defined as "sexist" because of his raw celebration of sexuality and his extranaked attention to female bodies, proves to be much more cunning than is ordinarily assumed when one carefully reads not just his body language (and his music videos) but also his lyrics. His sensitivity to the plight of disempowered woman and his advocacy of egalitarian gender relations, particularly in matters of sexual politics, are truly remarkable. Conversely, Bob Marley, in his smugly patriarchal Rastafari way, is potentially much more sexist than Shabba Ranks.

In chapter 3, "Lady Saw Cuts Loose: Female Fertility Rituals in the Dancehall," I argue that the celebration of the female body that is ritualized in the supposedly "secular" sphere of the dance may also be read as a sign of the continuity of West African traditions of embodied spirituality in the diaspora. Furthermore, the female DJ, having upstaged her male counterpart and taken control of the mike, assumes the power to represent herself verbally and dance to her own beat. But, somewhat paradoxically, she often speaks the very same sexually explicit body language as the male DJs, causing shortsighted detractors to dismiss her as being even more culpable than they—and the women in the audience who take vicarious pleasure in her daring self-exposure. Though seemingly complicit in her objectification, the self-assertive female DJ does speak back to the male, challenging many of the chauvinist limitations that are imposed on her gender.

Norman Stolzoff, like Iris Myrie, takes strong exception to my reading of dancehall culture as a potentially liberatory space for women. In yet another extended footnote, Stolzoff rehearses the conventional critique of dancehall culture as a discourse of commodification of women, stating the obvious: ". . . it is too simple to claim that slackness is necessarily liberatory."[38] Stolzoff fails to identify the source of that simpleminded opinion. But the context of his critique, starting with a reference to my work, implicates me in that assertion. I myself make no such claim that slackness is "necessarily liberatory." The liberation is contingent and oftentimes partial.

In "Slackness Hiding from Culture: Erotic Play in the Dancehall," I do argue that some of the DJs' lyrics "celebrate the economic and sexual independence of women, thus challenging the conservative gender ideology that is at the heart of both pornographic and fundamentalist conceptions of woman as commodity, virgin and whore."[39] But I also document some instances, with particular reference to Yellow Man, in which, for me, "the commodification of women's sexuality by men assumes truly vulgar proportions. . . . Woman is reduced to a collection of body parts which seem to function independent of her will."[40] I further argue in that early essay that ". . . even Yellowman's narrow sexism can be viewed somewhat expansively, especially by feminists who theorise the conjunction of gender, class and race, as a 'small man' revolt against the institutionalisation of working-class female domestic rule and middle/upper-class male dominance in Jamaican society. . . . [D]isempowered working-class men cannot be simply stigmatised and dismissed as unqualified 'oppressors' of women. Their own oppression by gender-blind classism and notions of matriarchy itself motivates their attempted oppression of women."[41]

Following Henry Louis Gates Jr.'s reading of Esu in *The Signifying Monkey*, I propose that the trickster figure Anansi "provides a West African model of 'wholeness' that transcends the polarities (en)gendered in Western cultures."[42] I further argue that "the Culture/Slackness antinomy extends beyond the domain of the half-heartedly suppressed 'vulgarity' of the DJ. Its culturally specific manifestations in Jamaica suggest not only the continuity of West African ideological traditions in the diaspora, but also the conflict between those traditions and the official Christian morality of the Garden of Eden in which both the suppression of sexuality and the secondariness of woman are institutionalised: Adam (and Eve) hiding from God: versus Esu as the gateway to God."[43]

Stolzoff, somewhat like Anansi whom he cites in his critique of my reading of slackness in the dancehall, appropriates the essence of my argument—first misrepresenting it, then claiming the "revised version" as his own. But Stolzoff is an inept Anansi who has not mastered the duplicitous arts of conceit. I find it odd that he uses a 1994 article, "Dancing Around Development," written for a popular audience and published in the *Sistren* newsletter, as the apparent basis on which to generalize about my work on this subject. He does not cite in his dismissive footnote quoted above my 1989-1990 essay, "Slackness Hiding from Culture: Erotic Play in the Dancehall," which much more amply represents my position. Be that as it may, it appears to me that Stolzoff is both misrepresenting and regurgitating my own argument in the following passage—without even a gesture towards its origin:

> What Cooper's analysis fails to capture is the true dynamic tension between culture and slackness. The role of the slack DJ is like that of Anancy, the trickster spider of Afro-Jamaican folklore, who turns the prideful seriousness of the strong back on itself through mockery. Slackness is a corrective to the stultifying sense of order and moral virtue that sometimes overtakes dancehall culture. On the other hand, culture provides a framework for social order that would prevent slackness from destroying all sense of right and wrong action. When Cooper advocates for slackness from a middle-class position, she misses a real opportunity to critique dancehall's excesses, both in its culture and slackness guises, and to identity truly liberatory trends in lyrical creativity.[44]

In chapter 4, "'Mama, Is That You?': Erotic Disguise in the Films *Dancehall Queen* and *Babymother*," I extend the analysis of the representations of female identity in dancehall culture by examining the fictional constructions of motherhood on the larger-than-life stage of the screen. *Dancehall Queen,* set in Jamaica, and *Babymother,* set in the United Kingdom, both contest notions of motherhood that attempt to imprison women indefinitely in roles of subservience within the domestic sphere, thus masking their full potential. Both films illustrate the struggle of these female protagonists to claim the right to exposure in the public space of the dance. Both Anita and Marcia desire to become "visible" and thus be acknowledged for their talent as DJ and Queen of the Dance respectively.

I must thank my colleague Jane Bryce, of the Cave Hill campus of the University of the West Indies, for asking a fundamental question when I first presented this paper in 2000 at our annual conference on West Indian Literature, held in Guyana. She wondered, and I paraphrase her, whether the masses of the people who attend the dancehall would share my interpretation of the meaning of the films. Widening the frame of reference beyond the immediate context of the dancehall, I expansively deconstructed that provocative question as an interrogation of the capacity of working-class people, in particular, and Jamaicans, in general, to philosophize about the meaning of our lives. For the dancehall is not a closed space; its borders are porous. All kinds of people come and go across its stage performing a variety of identities with varying degrees of sophistication. Indeed, playing *mas* is not the same as *not* knowing who you really are.

On later reflection it occurred to me that my colleague's skeptical question could also be decoded as a challenge to the cultural critic to provide "authoritative" readings of contested texts, authority having shifted from the academy to the street. The conventional function of the critic as interpreter of cultural meanings is thus subsumed in the new role of ventriloquist, projecting meanings that originate outside the academy. In theory, this is all very well and good in these postmodernist times. In practice, in my own work on Jamaican popular culture, I also claim for the critic a function of mediating. That mediation is not a distortion of meaning. Rather, it is a translation of the language of the street into the argot of the academy. More important, mediation is also a process of expanding the lexicon and grammar of academic discourse.

In chapter 5, "'Lyrical Gun': Metaphor and Role-Play in Dancehall Culture," I turn from the representations of permissive sexuality that are associated almost exclusively with female identity to an analysis of the construction of masculinity within discourses of violence that make the phallus and the gun synonymous. Arguing that the language of dancehall lyrics encodes elements of verbal play, especially braggadocio, and cannot always be taken literally, I focus on Buju Banton's infamous antihomosexuality song, "Boom By-By," emphasizing the metaphorical nature of the inflammatory discourse. On the locally produced 45 rpm record, the spelling of the song's title is "Boom By-By," representing the sound of gunfire. The song does not appear on any of Buju's own CDs, as far as I can tell. On a later compilation CD, the 'e' is added, thus reinforcing the final farewell of death.[45] For political reasons I privilege the original spelling.

In this chapter I also examine the ideological implications of marketing dancehall lyrics internationally—outside of the immediate context of primary cultural production and meaning. I pay attention to the resulting sound clashes that do occur when indigenous Jamaican/dancehall values cross borders and enter cultural spaces that cannot accommodate them. I coin the term "heterophobia" as a politically neutral label for a whole range of anxieties that plague all peoples in all cultures: phobias that are reducible to the singular *fear of difference*. Differences of race, ethnicity, gender, class, age and sexual orientation all generate phobias. "Heterophobia" is not the straight "opposite" of homophobia; it is an inclusive, generic designation whose multiple applications incorporate the current definitions of homophobia. Heterophobia goes straight to the heart of the problem of cultural difference.

My explication of the multivocal meaning of Buju Banton's song itself generated yet another sound clash with another North American academic. Like Norman Stolzoff, Andrew Ross, professor of American Studies at New York University, attempts to demonstrate the limitations of my argument on precisely this point of the cultural relativity of the insider's versus the outsider's reading of Jamaican popular culture. The particular issue at stake is the caveat I offer in the concluding paragraph of an early version of chapter 5, which was published in a special issue of the *Massachusetts Review* on Caribbean culture, edited by Rhonda Cobham-Sander. With respect to "Boom By-By" and, more generally, public discourse on homosexuality in Jamaica, I argue that "given the historical context of a dislocating politics of Euro-American imperialism in the region, 'hard-core' Jamaican cultural nationalists are likely to resist any re-examination of indigenous values that is perceived as imposed on them by their imperial neighbour in the North."[46]

In his intriguing essay, "Mr. Reggae DJ, Meet the International Monetary Fund," Ross first misquotes my statement: My speculative "are likely to resist" becomes his authoritative "will resist."[47] To some readers there may be no difference between the two statements, but my intention was to suggest possibilities rather than to predict outcomes. Further, Ross concludes that my caveat "illustrates the chronic conflict between the universal assumptions of northern liberal conceptions of human rights and the culturally specific assumptions of southern countries."[48] His cunning syntax here engenders ambiguities. Does Ross mean that liberal northerners erroneously assume that what are really their own culture-specific conceptions are universal norms; and that southerners sensibly assume that their conceptions are not universal but culture specific? Or does he mean that "universal . . . human rights" is a uniquely northern liberal preoccupation and that the inhumane South remains silent on this issue in its cultural specificity? Which brings us to that chronically troubling "universal"/"culturally specific" opposition. Supposedly "universal" assumptions often manifest themselves in very culture-specific ways. Some cultures are a priori "universal" and others never achieve universality, however hard (or little) they try. In addition, my "imperial" is transmuted into Ross's "universal." But, perhaps, in some quarters those words are synonymous.

Furthermore, Ross fails to quote in its entirety the conclusion to my essay in which I make it absolutely clear that Jamaican society is undergoing fundamental change on the contentious matter of homosexuality. In this instance, Ross's tendentious assertions about the apparent fixity of the "culturally specific assumptions of southern countries" are decidedly invalidated. Indeed, the sentence that Ross does quote actually begins with a "however" that he omits; the elision thus conceals the relationship between the quoted passage and that which precedes it: "The international marketing of reggae is raising fundamental questions about cultural identity, cultural autonomy and the right to cultural difference. On the issue of sexual preference, Jamaican society is itself slowly moving in the direction of giving visible cultural space to homosexuals. However, given the historical context of a dislocating politics of euro-american imperialism in the region, 'hard-core' Jamaican cultural nationalists are likely to resist any re-examination of indigenous values that is perceived as imposed on them by their imperial neighbour in the North."[49]

Headstrong, Ross insistently attempts to undermine my presumably nonuniversal southern assumptions and, accordingly, fails to acknowledge my own recognition of the complexity of the cultural transactions that take place across North/South borders:

> But Cooper's argument that "politically correct" northern liberalism is continuous with classic colonialist patterns is worth examining further, especially in light of the new cultural patterns produced by a globalizing economy.
>
> Cooper's recognition of the strict opposition between local and foreign values does not necessarily do justice to competing forms of nationalism within the postcolonial state, nor does it address the complex moral geography that links Caribbean states with the immigrant-busy metropoles.[50]

First of all, as Stuart Hall reminds us, "globalization must never be read as a simple process of cultural homogenization; it is always an articulation of the local, of the specific and the global." But, in any case, as I explicitly state in the *Massachusetts Review* article:

> The politics of representation are complicated: it would appear that homosexuals in Jamaica themselves accept the social contract—proverbially expressed, that "where ignorance is bliss, tis folly to be wise." Coming out leaves no room for blissful ignorance of one's sexual preference. It allows no

uncontested space for role play. Migration from the closed, heterophobic world of Jamaican society does facilitate less ambiguous modes of self-representation. For example, it is rumoured in Jamaica that the lyrics of "Boom By-By" were translated for GLAAD by a migrant Jamaican homosexual living in New York. This collaboration of North American and Jamaican homosexuals marks a new stage of politicisation of consciousness outside of, and within Jamaica, around issues of heterophobia.[51]

It seems to me that even if my argument here does not explicitly take up the issue of "competing forms of nationalism within the postcolonial state," it nevertheless does "address the complex moral geography that links Caribbean states with the immigrant-busy metropoles." My "complicated" becomes Ross's "complex"; my "migrant Jamaican" becomes his "immigrant busy metropoles"; my "new stage of politicization" becomes his "moral geography." But perhaps my southern propensities make it impossible for me to recognize the world of difference between the sophisticated insights of this liberal northern academic and my presumably simpleminded, culturally specific, insular truisms.

An early version of Andrew Ross's contentious argument appears in an embryonic paper, "The Structural Adjustment Blues," presented at an international conference on Caribbean culture hosted by the University of the West Indies, Mona, Jamaica in 1996. I challenged him in private on the matter of his oversimplification of my reading of the politics of migration. He conceded that my argument was, indeed, more subtle than his account of it. Nevertheless, he willfully reproduced, embellished even, the misreading in this twice-published paper. I expect that he knows that not many of his readers will bother to check my article to see what I actually say; they will simply take his word for it. Furthermore, in footnote 16 of "Mr. Reggae DJ, Meet the International Monetary Fund," Ross rightly declares that "[t]here is virtually no literature on homosexuality in Jamaica." I was, therefore, surprised to discover that he fails to indicate any source for the information he provides in the very sentence that he *does* footnote: ". . . working-class queers are often street higglers or vendors, giving back as good as they get in the way of verbal banter and abuse."[52] This assertion seems remarkably similar to the statement I myself make in "'Lyrical Gun'" that "clearly 'out' male homosexuals work as higglers in Jamaican markets and ply their trade with relatively little provocation. Many have mastered the art of 'tracing'—ritualized verbal abuse—as a form of protection from the heterophobia of Jamaican society."[53] Coming from the North, Ross can be confident that his scholarship is unquestionable and his authority is assured.

Incidentally, Ross enthuses thus in the blurb to Stolzoff's book on Jamaican sound systems: "This is the first sustained study of Jamaican dancehall music and culture in all its aspects. Everyone interested in the island music, and in popular music in general, will find something useful in this book." But, as I have argued, a major aspect of dancehall music and culture is the meaning of lyrics, a subject that Stolzoff dismisses as having relatively little value. Citing Paul Gilroy, the don of "black atlantic" studies, who, in turn, cites the even bigger don of "white atlantic" studies, Michel Foucault, Stolzoff takes comfort in the delusion that he himself is not "caught up in the textual, semiotic level of analysis."[54] But even Stolzoff's "nonlyrical" anthropological analysis is indeed "textual" and "semiotic" and, in its own way, reduces the "open hazardous reality of conflict [in dancehall culture]" to the "calm Platonic form of language and dialogue [in his book]"—to cite Stolzoff, citing Gilroy, citing Foucault.[55]

Although Stolzoff disdains lyrical analysis, he is forced, on occasion, to pay attention to the verbal artistry of the DJs/selectors in order to reinforce his own argument about the total meaning of dancehall performance. Indeed, the opening pages of his preface vividly document the verbal ricochet that is the sound system clash: "The song's first line carries the audience away in a burst of enthusiasm. Cigarette lighters flash, rags wave, whistles shrill, hands thrust upward, legs kick out, voices curse with joy. Standing in the eye of the storm, Trooper attempts to maintain his composure, but he is obviously delighted. 'Hear this,' he bellows over the booming record."[56] In effect, Stolzoff's account of what he is doing in his own book often clashes with his actual practice. Proverbial wisdom in Jamaica warns, "finger never seh 'look ya,' it always seh 'look deh." [The pointing finger never says "look here," it always says "look there."] The point of the proverb, at the literal level, is that the thumb always focuses inward on the speaker even as the index finger moves outward to indicate/ indict the other. Metaphorically, the proverb warns of the danger of failing to acknowledge one's own vulnerability even as one points out the failings of others. I myself am ever mindful of this warning.

In addition, Andrew Ross, writing out of his own cultural specificities, does not appear to know how much the generic "island" label irks many Caribbean peoples whose cultural specificity is thus erased. An apostrophe s—"the island's music"—would have made all the difference in how the touristy/world beat "island music" category is received by some Caribbean readers. The Antiguan novelist Jamaica Kincaid gives a biting critique of the casually homogenizing "island" imperative in her novel *Lucy*. In the words of the protagonist: "I had met Dinah the night after we arrived here on our holiday, and I did not like her. This was because the first thing she said to me when Mariah introduced us was 'So you are from the islands?' I don't know why, but the way she said it made a fury rise up in me. I was about to respond to her in this way: 'Which islands exactly do you mean? The Hawaiian Islands? The islands that make up Indonesia or what?' And I was going to say it in a voice that I hoped would make her feel like a piece of nothing, which was the way she had made me feel in the first place."[57]

In chapter 6, "'More Fire': Chanting down Babylon from Bob Marley to Capleton," I again invoke the iconic status of Bob Marley in order to challenge the popular misconception that there is an insurmountable ideological divide between the culture of reggae and its dancehall off-spring. Focusing on the metaphor of fire, I establish the genealogical link between the lyrical representation of old and new Rastafari discourses and demonstrate the ways in which Capleton's incendiary dancehall *riddims* echo Bob Marley's equally inflammatory rhythms of resistance against the system. I do recognize differences in the tone and temper of the lyrics of both artists. Nevertheless, I focus on the similarities that are so often overlooked in dismissive evaluations of the "degeneracy" of contemporary dancehall music.

In chapter 7, "'Vile Vocals': Exporting Jamaican Dancehall Lyrics to Barbados," as in chapter 6, I document some of the sound clashes that do occur when Jamaican dancehall culture crosses borders and takes root in the eastern Caribbean, especially in a seemingly conservative society like Barbados. "Vile Vocals: Unofficial War in Bim" is the headline of an April 11, 2000, editorial published in the national newspaper, the *Barbados Advocate,* which articulates not only the contempt with which the lyrics themselves are vilified by the "status crow," to cite Kamau Brathwaite's subversion of status quo; but also the disdain that my ameliorative reading of the discourse engenders.

In its continued campaign to keep "little England" safe from vile influences, the *Barbados Advocate* published on June 23, 2002, a fascinating letter attributed to one Mrs. Corneldi Watts from Montego Bay, Jamaica, headlined "Ban the nasty lyrics."[58] This impassioned opinion piece amply expresses practically every stereotype about Jamaican dancehall culture: DJs "can barely read or write"; their "message" is "generally negative and violent"; their repertoire consists of "derogatory, women degrading, sexually explicit songs"; their "'music' is just loud and boisterous cackling, oftentimes unintelligible and offensive to the ear"; the dancehall is a quintessentially violent space where "nine times out of ten at these bashments, a fight will break out and people will be killed"; DJs are "criminals," "sellers of songs 'bigging up' drugs, sex and murder!" It is instructive to note how sex here is so casually criminalized along with drugs and murder.

Not surprisingly, given the context in which her letter is published, Watts makes an uncharitable comparison between dancehall and soca, misrepresenting the multifaceted eastern Caribbean music as purely "wave yuh flag," happy-go-lucky party music. All of the social commentary in soca is repressed as well as the salacious double entendres that confirm the music's kinship with dancehall slackness. Soca is reconstituted as fundamentally different in ethos from its Jamaican dancehall variant. Watts concludes her letter by invoking "wonderful Bob Marley," thus underscoring the contrast between dancehall music and not just soca, but also "real" Jamaican popular music of yore:

> Fool yourself not. Soca is a delightful form of music and is nothing like the garbage that they sing, which seems to be a common line used in their defense. Nothing is as dirty and awful as what Jamaica has to offer in the 21st century in terms of music.
>
> Suddenly, the wonderful *Bob Marley* and others of that era seem a hundred years ago. God help you Barbados, if you weaken and give in to the criminals calling themselves "singers."
>
> I am a sickened Jamaican.

In chapter 8, "Hip-hopping across Cultures: Reggae to Rap and Back," I examine the genealogical ties between dancehall and rap, yet another stigmatized African diasporic music. Watts's assertion that "[n]othing is as dirty and awful as what Jamaica has to offer in the 21st century in terms of music" would, I think, be vigorously challenged by those detractors of rap who claim that place of dishonor for this African American strain of contemporary Black music. Focusing on language and ideology, I draw attention to some of the similarities between the two musics, foregrounding the shared history of resistance to the dehumanizing definitions of African diasporic identities in the Americas.

In chapter 9, "'Mix Up the Indian with All the Patwa': Rajamuffin Sounds in Cool Britannia," I acknowledge the contribution of all those non-Jamaican DJs who have successfully reproduced the language and *riddims* of the dancehall: Nahki in Japan, Snow in Canada. Bigga Haitian in New York, Admiral T in Guadeloupe, Gentleman in Germany, to name just a few of the non-Jamaican artists who have DJed across cultural borders and mastered the sound clash on home territory and internationally. Their accomplishment is a compelling confirmation of the seductive power of Jamaican dancehall culture and its infinite capacity for adaptation. In particular, I pay attention to the work of Apache Indian, who was born in Birmingham, United Kingdom and there learned the complex modes of self-representation as a "Jamaican" dancehall DJ. Apache Indian DJs like a native. And, indeed, Birmingham—especially the Handsworth district—is very much a Jamaican city, providing the Black British DJ with role models of performative excellence within a distinctly Caribbean idiom. Having appropriated the "patwa" language of Jamaicans in the United Kingdom, Apache mixes this with the Punjabi he learned at home. What results is a polyvocal, rajamuffin sound that noises abroad the multiculti ethos of Tony Blair's "cool" Britannia. Apache Indian himself concedes that his experiment also confirms the problematic politics of "acculturation" in communities of mutual suspicion.

In the concluding chapter, "The Dancehall Transnation: Language, Lit/orature, and Global Jamaica," Hubert Devonish and I analyze the central role of "patwa," the language of choice for local DJs and their foreign imitators, in defining a truly populist and inter/national Jamaican identity. Beginning with an examination of eighteenth-century texts, we document the history of sound clashes in Jamaica between competing definitions of national identity, articulated in the dissonance between English and "patwa" discourses. In "postcolonial" Jamaica, language still functions to define insiders and outsiders, the civilized and the barbaric. Much of the contempt that the DJs attract is a consequence of their celebration of their mother tongue, Jamaican, as the natural language of artistic performance. But, somewhat ironically, it is this very language, carried abroad with such consummate ease by Jamaican musicians over the last four decades, that has helped to consolidate a global identity for the brand name Jamaica.

ONE

Border Clash

Sites of Contestation

(co-author Cecil Gutzmore)

Yu know dem send fi di Don inna di border clash

[You know they sent for the Don at the border clash][1]

—Ninjaman, "Border Clash"

Ninjaman's 1990 composition "Border Clash" is the classic articulation of a recurring motif in Jamaican dancehall culture that demarcates contestations for power in a wide range of spheres of influence. In its narrowest sense, the dancehall clash denotes the onstage competition between rival DJs and sound systems contending for mastery before a discriminating audience. More broadly, the clash is not just the performance event but becomes a trenchant metaphor for the hostile interfacing of warring zones in Jamaican society where, for example, rival politicians, area dons/community leaders, and their followers contend for the control of territory, both literal and symbolic. Its meaning thus widened, the dancehall trope of the "border clash" ultimately speaks to ideological conflicts between competing value systems in Jamaica.

Ninjaman composed "Border Clash" in the heat of battle at a celebrated show, billed as a "Border Clash," and staged at a venue—the now-defunct Coney Park—that was literally on the borderline between St. Catherine and St. Andrew/Kingston. Donna Hope gives a vivid eyewitness account of the event in her insightful Master's thesis:

> The deejays billed, including Ninjaman and Admiral Bailey from Kingston versus artistes like Papa San, Skullman and up and coming no-names from St. Catherine, created high levels of expectation in the Border Clash audience. These expectations were not met as, up until midnight, not one single high-ranking artiste had graced the stage. The poorly organized event had suffered lengthy stage preparations and band set-up and the Master of Ceremonies, Richie B, had been hard-pressed to contain the burgeoning frustration of the audience. As the screeching, off-key singing of Little Cherry gave way to another encore performance of a group of old men billed as the Skattalites, frustration ruptured through the audience. *Wi want big artiste. Ninja and Admiral. Wi tiyad a dis foolishness. [We want popular artists. Ninjaman and Admiral Bailey. We are tired of this foolishness.]* [2]

The organizers of the event must take full responsibility for the deterioration of the show into a clash with their frustrated patrons. Demanding audiences that pay for entertainment with hard-earned dollars have every right to expect good value for money. If this contract is breached by unscrupulous promoters and incompetent performers, disgusted patrons often assume the right to take matters into their own hands, quite literally. In an immediately effective form of communal critical judgment, the crowd often hurls missiles at "eedyat" (idiot) singers/DJs who have not mastered their craft, thus cruelly exercising the right to insist on high artistic standards.

This is precisely what happened at the "Border Clash" fiasco, as Hope recounts in exacting detail:

The first Shandy bottle ricocheted off the stage. Richie B's attempts to stem the tide was [*sic*] met with more Shandy bottles pelting the stage and, dodging one such missile, he beat a hasty retreat backstage. Derek, the bassmaster of Saggitarius [*sic*] band abandoned the stage and rushed after Richie B. Suddenly, all hands were picking up and hoisting Shandy bottles towards the deserted stage in a veritable rain of glass. It was Ninjaman who saved the day. Secure in his identification as the master of Clash and the ultimate Don Gorgon he hastily strode on stage holding his left hand aloft and palm outwards in a commanding and placatory gesture—"Hooold on"—and instantly transformed the violent mood of the crowd into one of exultation and celebration. His lengthy performance of nearly two hours effectively stemmed the flow of audience-stage real violence and transformed this into a celebration of lyrical violence.[3]

In the case of Ninjaman's apparently spontaneous composition, "Border Clash," the melodramatic confrontation between performer and audience on aesthetic grounds becomes instantly transmuted into pure theater: "phenomenon one." The latter phrase, a favorite of Ninjaman's, not only denotes his prodigious talent as a master of the art of DJing—in the colloquial sense of "phenomenon"—but also incorporates the philosophical meaning of the word: "that of which the senses or the mind directly takes note; an immediate object of perception," to cite the *Oxford English Dictionary (OED)* definitions. Indeed, Ninjaman's creative act of DJing about the immediate object of his perception at the show—the audience's rage—exemplifies his characteristically intelligent response to the particular circumstances of each event at which he performs. In a telephone conversation Ninjaman reflected thus on his strategy: "Mi performance build off a show an di spirit weh me see a gwaan" [My performance takes its structure from the event itself and from the spirit I feel there].[4]

Using his own verbal skill to defuse the hostility of the crowd, and, indeed, to unite the audience in celebration of his talent, Ninjaman grandly demonstrated at the "Border Clash" event that he, "the original front teet[h], gold teet, Don Gorgon," was the real master of the Clash. He cunningly asserts that there was, indeed, no competition—for him—at the alleged Clash. Line by line, the DJ gives a compelling account of how to avoid defeat in the lyrical battle of wits. Ninjaman's vivid image of lining out lyrics cleverly denotes both the metrical line of his verse as well as the overall linear narrative structure of the rhythmic tale he tells.

Recalling the 1990 affair more than a decade later, Ninjaman humorously observed, "Mi ha fi find a way fi mek no bockle no fling pon mi, so mi ha fi defend di two side" [I had to find a way to avoid being hit by bottles so I had to defend both sides].[5] These two sides were, primarily, the supporters of the clashing DJs from Kingston and St. Catherine; but as Ninjaman makes clear in the song, the two sides did collaborate to vent their collective anger at the poor performances from the opening acts. The DJ delineates the painful circumstances in which incompetent performers are routinely forced to flee from the stage: hit by weapons of mass destruction. Angry performers have been known to return fire at the crowd amassed against them.

Despite the hard evidence of bottle, stone, and the flying bullet of the gunshot salute, the violence in the Jamaican dancehall is primarily verbal. Indeed, it is the performer's facility with words that is contested in this domain. A spectacular exception to this rule is the much lamented fist fight between Ninjaman and newcomer Vybz Kartel that erupted at Sting 2003, in violation of the conventions of the clash. All of the DJs routinely engage in verbal confrontation, pitting wits and lyrics against each other. The metaphorical nature of much of this discourse—for example, the gun talk—is usually lost on narrow-minded critics of the genre who fail to understand the element of play in the language of the dancehall and thus take the DJs' lyrics all too literally. In this sportive spirit of braggadocio, Ninjaman strategically detonates his lyrical bombs and artfully discharges his figurative arsenal of guns in "Border Clash" in order to bring down the house. The Jamaican creole expression "tear down the house" and its variant, "mash up the place," are the exact equivalent of the English "bring down the house," as defined by the *OED:* "to evoke applause which suggests the downfall of the building." The more vigorous Jamaican metaphors, with their overtones of "violence," are just as figurative as their English counterpart.

The response of the audience, Ninjaman declares, is an ecstatic gun salute to the explosive lyrics he draws from his storehouse of words. The DJ's use of "draw" here primarily denotes the pulling out of the gun; but it simultaneously connotes Ninjaman's drawing on his lyrical reserves to create rhyming words, rhythmic patterns and evocative metaphors that the audience will validate as appropriately "dangerous." The latter word, like the African American "bad," subversively signals an ironic inversion of values and the concomitant intensity of pleasure that the DJ's boastful talk of badness elicits.

Indeed, despite all of the lyrical gunfire, Ninjaman ends "Border Clash" with an exhortation to good citizenship that would surprise those outsiders who do not understand the multi-track discourse of the dance-hall, as the following anecdote illustrates. Invited in October 2002 to give a talk in the Reggae Studies lecture series at the University of the West Indies, Mona, Jamaica, the DJ chose as the title of his presentation, "Ninjaman's Programme to Elevate Jamaica." Skeptics questioned his capacity to speak with authority on the subject. Decent citizens bombarded the University administration with strident complaints that the decision to invite the DJ to lecture was a clear sign that the walls of the ivory tower had been irreparably breached. On Friday, October 13, the *Daily Observer* converted into national news a routine press release announcing the DJ's presentation.

Ninjaman did not keep the engagement. In response, the October 15 *Sunday Observer* published a mischievous cartoon: a notice on the chalkboard in a lecture room, presumably on the campus of the University of the West Indies, Mona, announces Ninjaman's talk, scheduled for 5:00 P.M. A clock says 7:00 P.M. The teacher looks impatiently at her watch. Two students are fast asleep and one of the remaining two says to her, "Him not coming again Miss Cooper, maybe him gone border clash." [He's not coming after all Miss Cooper; perhaps he's gone to a border clash.] The derisory cartoon does not at all accurately reflect what happened. A capacity audience of over three hundred students, faculty, and members of the public engaged in lively conversation about the meaning of Ninjaman's work when it became clear that he was not going to appear. I led the discussion that lasted for well over an hour.

The following week Ninjaman did talk at the University, functioning as the opening act for Louise Frazer-Bennett. He offered an apology for his no-show and promised to return to elaborate his program to elevate the country: "Jamaica a go dung into a pothole. And we need . . . not me, not you, not just some of us . . . we need the whole country to come together and mek a start. The Prime Minister himself need help." [Jamaica is going down into a pothole. And we need . . . not me, not you, not just some of us . . . we need the whole country to come together and start all over. The Prime Minister himself needs help]. Ninjaman's vivid metaphor of the state machinery crashing in a pothole effectively trans- mutes the mundane horrors of Jamaica's roads into the symbolic lan- guage of lyrical inventiveness.

The DJ himself thus acknowledges in "Border Clash" that his bad- man gun talk is pure badinage, a grand rhetorical performance. He urges the audience to decode his encrypted message: the only way that condi- tions in Jamaica will improve is if love, harmony, and unity prevail. Ninjaman asserts that the dancehall has the potential to become a unifying space in which skanking [dancing] is the great social leveler. In "Border Clash," Ninjaman himself skanks effortlessly between the literal and the metaphorical; between the sounds of war and the rhetoric of peace.

Taken out of the immediate context of the dancehall event, the concept "border clash" has resonance in defining a broad range of conflicts in Jamaican society. Contested borders are located across language barriers (English versus Jamaican); Jamaican Creole is the language of the popular, especially that of the DJs. It defines itself against and clashes with English—still the singular language of elitist national identity in Jamaica and, thus, of all official discourse. There are also sound clashes between cultural genres and their related practices (reggae versus dancehall; and both versus soca/carnival). There are contestations between social spaces ("ghetto" versus "uptown"). There are clashes of interests such as those of the "politician" and "ghetto youths." There is competition between pigment shades ("Black woman" versus "browning"—Jamaican slang for mulatto hybridity). Female rivals competing for the attention, affection, and material resources of shared male lovers give new meaning to erogenous zones, which are redefined as zones of warfare. Eros and Mars clashing, as it were, for the right to reign as supreme champion.

Border clashes occur between religious positions: for example, Rastafari versus Christianity, particularly the Roman Catholic Church, which is identified in popular discourse with the biblical beast of St. John's apocalypse. Border clashes also manifest themselves within Rastafari between the House of the Bobo Dreads of Prince Emmanuel and all other houses. This is one of the most intriguing of the ongoing border clashes within the Jamaican popular. The Bobo Dreads represent Rastafari's closest connection to the very bottom stratum of Jamaican society. Wishing to elevate the children of Africa, they use royal titles such as king, queen, prince, and princess in addressing fellow Africans, and they have popularized a new Rastafari salutation, "Blessed/Blessed love." Their main camp under their now ancestor leader, Prince Emmanuel Edwards, is outside Kingston at Bull Bay, and followers have created another nucleus in August Town, on the Hope River, center of the movement of the early twentieth-century charismatic leader Alexander Bedward and site of his famed "healing stream." Here in August Town the Rastafari DJ Sizzla has his home base.

The Bobo Dreads have conceived an original theology in which Prince Emmanuel himself, Haile Selassie, and Marcus Garvey appear as a trinity of deities. The theological and social doctrines of the Bobo Dreads are rejectionist and radical. For example, in the 2003 Trevor Rhone film, *One Love,* the hard-line Bobo Dred musician is the most vociferous antagonist of the Christian young woman who wins the heart of the lead singer Rastaman. Christian theology is repudiated by the Bobos, if not in total, then very nearly so. Jesus is not deified, and his relationship with his disciples is interpreted as involving homosexual practice. This may represent the harder Bobo position; a softer, more subtle one claims to be attacking not the actual *Jessus Christus* but the false white image of the celebrated Michelangelo painting, "The Last Supper." The Bobos chant up sounds directed at "cleansing and purifying" not just the doctrines of Rastafari but also Jamaican society more widely. Their anathema against what they see as "corruption" requires invocation of divine "fire bun" [burning fire] to consume the offending entity, which may be person, thing, practice, or even other deity. There are reports of a certain willingness on the part of some Bobos to use more than verbal violence against representatives of other Houses of Rastafari and non-Rastafari.

Clashes between competing bodies of Rastafari and contradictory definitions of Rastafari doctrine and *livity* are not at all peculiar to the contemporary moment. There is a long history of contestation between various groups struggling to claim and name divinity. A 1971 missive written by Ras Dizzy, "Poet, Artist and Black Writer," as he describes himself, is a classic manifestation of this "discord and division."[6] Cunningly headlined "CONDEMN NONE SAYETH THE LORD, LESS YOU SHALL BE CONDEMNED," the letter nevertheless is a damning account of Ras Dizzy's disaffection with the leadership of the Ethiopian Federation 15, more popularly known as the Twelve Tribes of Israel, whose leaders were based in East Kingston. The first paragraph of the letter is an excellent example of the rhetoric of mystical invective, worthy of full quotation—with its idiosyncratic punctuation, spelling, and diction all intact. Ras Dizzy begins with the disarming salutation, "Hello there

Readers, Peace and Love in the name of the most High God Rastafari," and immediately thereafter declares unequivocal war:

> Folks, this is important—A group of Rastas get together in speaking and self celebration at Glasspole Avenue in East Kingston on Sunday night, but I am afraid that only the colours of the Rainbow and some interpretation of the Bible included their apparels and precept, helps the company of this particular group, which is the Ethiopian Federation 15, that would give them any identity as true Rastafarians. It is a real self business set-up.

After that opening salvo, with its sardonic focus on the habits of deception, Ras Dizzy proceeds to itemize the failings of the narcissistic group, foregrounding the sound clash between those who call on the name of Jesus and those who hail Selassie:

> Firstly, to commence with, is that the cult who invited the rest of his Federation 15 group to this session is a liver in the Glasspole Avenue Community, and he does not even tell the other brethren around the said community about it, unless you was a member of that particular group. In the company of their self session then they started to make a division against the locksman who is the terrible and dreadful angel and prophet of the Almighty God—as I appeared in the audience I had greeted the Lion of Juda, Haile Selassie I, name by I hailing to the HolyGod and the Covenant of Creation, Rastafari. But before I could finish I was challenged by members of the group, when about 8 voices give out saying—"Is Jesus we deal with hereso"—and so from that moment on then it was discord and division—they talk to their other brethren who is not a member of the Ethiopian Federation 15 like dog—they even went more than that by telling the others that if you were not a member of their group you can't get to Ethiopia nor heaven. They cannot reason divinely, rationally nor with love, with dignity nor with peace. Some of their foolish and show-off followers

nearly get themselves killed off for they try to open violence in trying to force one to be a member of theirs, and to say Jesus, instead of Rastafari.

Ras Dizzy dismissively elaborates his disdain for those who, venerating the name of Jesus, "make a division against the locksman." He further identifies a broad range of inter/national religious and political institutions that are all branded with the name of Jesus:

> At that stage then, it should be made known that the name to the God Jesus, is the one which all the Babylonian Governant, servants and men, always from time to time worship in—and now the G.G. [Governor General, Representative of the Queen], the Prime Ministers, the Police, the False Judge, the P.M. of South Africa and as well, Rhodesia and the Pope of Rome, all bow down to this God, through the translation which came by Latin and Greek, fights against the true God and his true anointed prophet and saints. It is for these true factors why Shadrack, Meishoc and Abendigo was thrown into the fire—Daniel into the Lions Den—and too the beheading of John the Baptist.

Ras Dizzy concludes his missive with an appeal to unity, emphasizing his own ability to tolerate diverse opinions without resorting to abuse:

> When I addressed over 800 students including the other accompanying crowd, I had dispute and contrary reflections, but I never insulted none, condemned none nor sayeth only Ras Dizzy and the T.F.R.C. [Triumphant Faith of the Rastafari Church] can go to Ethiopia. Anything forced one to join in is not proper—Who doesnot [sic] come to my group then I don't pass them on the street and malice them like a pagon [sic] would—it is time to stop this discordance among ourselves, because all who do such gets nowhere.

Contemporary hard-line Bobos are provoking a reaction expressed in the popular through a series of songs attempting to ridicule their alleged desire to "fire bun" everything. One such song is by no less a figure than Beenie Man, who alleged in a 1998 interview with Winford Williams, in the CVM Television "On Stage" series, that he had been assaulted by "some a Capleton man dem" at the Norman Manley airport. At the January 31, 1999, Ethiopian Orthodox Church service in honor of Bob Marley's fifty-fourth birthday, the sermon partly targeted Bobo attitudes. The self-styled prophet Capleton is certainly an articulate advocate of the Bobo position. So also is Sizzla and their message reverberates in the work of Anthony B, Junior Reed, Charley Chaplin, and many other youthful griots.

Border clashes are also evident in the host of encounters that take place between forces that can be categorized as "cultural imperialism" and those that are local and specific to Jamaican (popular) culture. For example, one of Jamaica's two national daily newspapers, the *Jamaica Observer,* carried in its weekend edition of March 6, 1998, a story headlined, "'Shiprider' takes effect Tuesday." This is a reference to the international agreement between Jamaica and the United States "to allow American ships and aircraft to enter the island's seas and airspace in pursuit of suspected drug traffickers."[7] This agreement has been strongly contested locally, even though the version signed by the government of Jamaica is somewhat less disempowering than that signed by its Eastern Caribbean neighbors. The potential for border clashes is disquieting in these problematic transactions that take place across the porous juridical boundaries of small-island states, menaced by global, multinational, and superpower forces.

The integrity of the juridical and cultural entity represented as "Jamaica" also is challenged in more intriguing ways. At the 1996 conference of the U.K. Society for Caribbean Studies, a Black British participant, Denise Noble, then a senior lecturer in social work and sociology at the University of East London, asked in response to our papers on Jamaican popular music if it was not "essentialist" to use the term "Jamaican" to describe dancehall, given the way reggae has developed internationally.

Similarly, in her essay "Ragga Music: Dis/Respecting Black Women and Dis/Reputable Sexualities," Noble observes, "To extend Cooper's analysis beyond a local Jamaican particularism, and questions of Jamaican national identity, we must engage with the diasporicity . . . of reggae music and reggae dancehall culture."[8]

Noble's question and its elaboration in the essay just cited seem to be overly influenced by "postmodernist" anxieties about nationalism and essentialism. Although it is true that Jamaican popular music has been dispersed globally—first, in the movement of Jamaican migrants to the United Kingdom, North America, and beyond; and, second, as part of the process of transnational capitalist consumerism—the essential character of the music, even in migration, owes much to its genesis and continuing reproduction in the Jamaican imaginary, shaped by culture-specific sociopolitical and economic realities, including racism, anticolonialism, and Black nationalism. Moreover, even in their Black British manifestations, reggae and ragga retain much of the radical political substance of their distinctive Jamaican origins, however mutated in the process of dispersal and re-creation. Scholarship driven by antiessentialist anxieties disregards precisely this kind of local cultural specificity.

Outside the boundary of the nation-state that is Jamaica is a vast territory variously termed "foreign," "far out," and "outernational." The words "far out" and "outernational" are examples of the way in which some Jamaican speakers reinterpret borrowed English words via folk etymology.[9] Words cross language barriers, assume new identities, and engender lexical and morphological clashes. The English word "foreign" is pronounced "farin" in Jamaican, consistent with a pattern of regular vowel change: from "o" to "a." Further, "foreign," which is monomorphemic in English, becomes reinterpreted as bimorphemic in Jamaican—"far" and "in." There is perceived to be a clash between the meaning of the word and the meaning of the "in" morpheme: "Farin" is "out," not "in." The "out" in "far out" thus aligns the meaning of the word and the meaning of the morpheme. In the case of the borrowed English word "international," "inter" is not recognized as a morpheme in Jamaican. But the "in" is. Again, a clash of meanings is perceived—"in" versus "out"—and "outernational" becomes the logical resolution.

This far/outer/national space holds terrors for those Jamaicans who try to cross legally and otherwise into lands of economic opportunity, particularly the United States and, less so, the United Kingdom. The first terror zone to be negotiated is the foreign embassy in Jamaica, where the quest for the elusive visa can assume Sisyphean proportions. Although the average Jamaican must jump through many hoops to get a visa, most reggae singers and DJs have relatively little difficulty getting past this barrier and negotiating their way through the maze of international travel. The music and its live performers have long gone "outernational." "Farin" contains, inter alia, friendly "massives"/"posses" in major cities of the world—London, Birmingham, New York, Hartford, Toronto, Cologne, Munich, Tokyo, Lagos, Accra, Harare, Sydney, Auckland, and so on. Performers credit these collectivities as constituting a global market that enables the artists to "break" or "bus" [burst] across national borders, or, as Shabba Ranks puts it, to "fly offa Jamaica map."[10]

These popular culture artists who so easily travel and sometimes "break big" outernationally can find that the "massive" there are as complex and as selective as those at home. As we say in Jamaican, "dem naa tek everyting" [they don't accept everything]. So a Buju and a Shabba Ranks run into trouble. They have border clashes with one increasingly empowered, if still heavily policed and sometimes silenced, outernational massive—the gay community—at the point at which the one sings "Boom By-By" and the other denounces gay people from his secular pulpit. Shabba is said to have "bowed"—succumbed to market forces and modified his message. But Buju is more assertively part of a movement at home that claims the right to denounce perceived wrongdoers.

For example, Terror Fabulous confidently declares that the righteous Rastaman will not be defeated in the war against the forces of darkness. Burning with the fire and brimstone of Old Testament authority, the DJ declares that Jah's soldiers, from east to west, will continue to increase into a formidable army that will never surrender.[11] Standing up for principle, the bonafide Rastaman, unlike the rent-a-dread facsimile, refuses to sell out. That vivid derisory metaphor, "rent-a-dread," signifies the dreadlock-sed pseudo Rasta, or Rastitute—the 'Rasta' prostitute who feeds off the sexual fantasies of both male and female tourists.

So Buju comes back stronger than ever, against blows aimed at him by the foreign and local Jamaican gay community, with the album *Till Shiloh,* especially the track "Complaint," featuring the late Garnet Silk. There is, too, the striking sight of Buju Banton bestride the pages of London's *The Guardian,* in its own way a shrine of outernational liberalism, a keeper of the gates of respectability. In an interview head-lined "A Roar from the Lion's Den," the DJ apparently disarms one of the paper's staffers, Kimi Zabihyan, converting the reporter into a channel through which his voice (supposedly dissonant in *Guardian* terms) is amplified: "On stage Buju prowls—and when I say like a lion he corrects me and says 'like a proud young lion,' stands up, trips over his rollerblade feet and pulls a face. At moments like this you remember that he's only 22" (that was in 1995).[12]

The captivating photograph of the DJ, which dominates the double-page text, is captioned thus: "Urban warrior . . . Buju Banton is a hero on the streets but remains tainted by his rampant homophobia." The headline encodes contradictions: the politically correct metaphor of the taint of homophobia, as well as the heroic image of the urban warrior. In that ambivalent moment, Buju, "determined to be heard," is given space to speak of the clashes of cultures on the borders of hetero/homosexuality, policed by the international media and capitalist record companies shor-ing up profits. Buju declares:

I was being heard before I was signed and I will continue. They brand Buju as preaching hostility to remove white people from listening to my music. The record companies want everything to coincide with their culture, but I

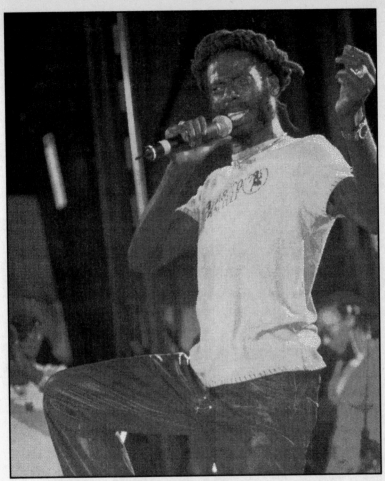

Buju Banton in performance at "Appleton Hotshots" in December 2003.
Photo: Carlington Wilmot.

say it's important for every culture to have its own road to travel on. In my culture, in African Caribbean culture, homosexuality is totally unacceptable. It's good when cultures meet but I have to deal with my people and stay true to my people. That is why I always kept my support, but even your enemy can do good for you. When they came out against Boom Bye Bye they drew attention to a poor ghetto youth. I'm an optimist.[13]

Buju Banton is the sort of optimist who understands what he's up against:

> "I want to know," asks Buju "do they sign us up or sign us off. They (the record companies) don't want to promote the authentic stuff. They want us to do this and that. Go with the reggae music I can't relate to, R&B or hip-hop. That isn't my culture. They want us to transform to cross-over. I want to reach people, but in crossing over we mustn't get lost. They want us to promote and sell their culture, but I won't cross over just to sell merchandise for other people."[14]

Those were Buju Banton's words while crossing the border between *Shiloh* and that new country with all those *Inna Heights* he reaches for and celebrates. The DJ unrepentantly asserts that it is culturally subversive authenticity that tears down the walls of Jericho and burns down Babylon, Sodom, and Gomorrah; that survives border clashes in this age of recolonizing globalization; that defeats capital's best efforts to transform counter-culture into "over-the-counter" culture.[15]

There are no easy victories to be scored in the border clash with heterosexism and homophobia of the type Buju Banton is undoubtedly representing. In this dangerous politics of location on the border, one does understand the cultural context out of which Buju speaks; at the same time, one must be prepared to fight for a much more progressive position on homosexuality on the very battleground that the DJ specifies as the African Jamaican cultural terrain. Indeed, Jamaican society is slowly transforming itself into a less repressive place for homosexuals. But the tradition of conservativism is deep-rooted. At the 1998 annual Boxing Day reggae extravaganza, Sting, a few weeks after the launching of the support group JFLAG, the Jamaican Forum for Lesbians, All-sexuals and Gays, Buju Banton began his set with the opening line of the infamous "Boom By-By." It was enough to put the crowd in an uproar. He did not even bother to perform the whole song. That solitary line was a potent statement of his refusal to bow at home to the pressures of what he perceives as external market forces.

A March 8, 1993, letter to the editor of the *Daily Gleaner*, entitled "Right to Hold Opinion," exemplifies the contradictory public response to homosexuality (and censorship of anti-homosexuality sentiment) in Jamaica. Written by a self-styled "Free Thinker," it was accorded "Letter of the Day" status by the newspaper. It is reproduced here in its entirety, punctuation errors and all:

> I understand that GLAAD, the homosexual group has local connections, so this letter may be of interest to them.
>
> The actions of their American and British counterparts against Buju Banton and Shabba Ranks and others, may be influencing people, but they are not winning any friends, especially not here in Jamaica.
>
> I hold no brief (pun intended) for either performer, as a matter of fact, my tastes in music run to jazz, the classics and oldies from the 1950s, 1960s and 1970s. However, I do defend the right of these performers to hold their own opinions.
>
> Homosexuals (I refuse to call nor consider them as "gay" as they seem a dour bunch) are, I believe, free to carry on their affairs as they see fit, so long as they keep it away from me. I find their sexual preference distasteful, to say the least. At the same time, I do not advocate violence against them and prefer the "live and let live" policy.
>
> On the other hand, whenever any interest group begins to attack the freedom of opinion and expression of others, there I draw a line.
>
> I would caution these members and supporters of GLAAD to watch out for the back lash that no doubt will eventually come, as many other persons are not as moderate as myself and they may see a resurgence of overt hostility from fans of these highly popular entertainers.

My advice to homosexuals is to feel pleased at your progress and increased acceptance but do not push your luck. Your continued freedom to enjoy your chosen lifestyle just may depend on your acceptance that not everyone shares your belief.[16]

This letter inscribes both the illusion of liberalism as well as a thinly veiled threat masquerading as "advice to homosexuals." It illustrates the schizophrenia of a sexually conservative society undergoing and resisting profound transformation.

In *Dangerous Crossroads: Popular Music, Postmodernism and the Poetics of Place,* professor of ethnic studies George Lipsitz argues:

The cross-cultural communication carried on within today's contemporary music retains residual contradictions of centuries of colonialism, class domination, and racism. But it also speaks to currents of culture and politics emerging from fundamentally new geopolitical and economic realities. The rapid mobility of capital and populations across the globe has problematized traditional understandings of place and made displacement a widely shared experience. Under these conditions, dispersed populations of migrant workers, emigrants, and exiles take on new roles as cross-cultural interpreters and analysts. As transnational corporations create integrated global markets and the nation state recedes as a source of identity and identification, popular culture becomes an ever more important public sphere.[17]

The "deportee," a volatile category of Jamaican migrant inscribed in popular music, is a classic example of the transgressive refugee who keeps crisscrossing national borders. "Deportees" are "yardies"—Jamaican citizens—who have fallen foul of overseas law enforcement agencies.

In a witty metaphorical transfer the word "deportee" in Jamaica also denotes a relatively cheap, reconditioned automobile, especially those originating in the Japanese domestic market. These secondhand vehicles have greatly increased the mobility of lower-income Jamaicans who cannot afford the higher-priced, export-market Japanese models. But they do have a whiff of illegality about them, somewhat like the moral odor that taints the human deportee. Insurance companies are becoming increasingly unwilling to insure these vehicles because they are perceived as high risk. For example, the relative unavailability of replacement parts means that in many instances the sum of the parts is decidedly more expensive than the whole car.

Human deportees may be repatriated on flights specially chartered for them. Or they take regular flights from cities like London. Under escort, these deportees, who are usually male, often cut a very sorry figure as they wait in the departure lounge. On arrival in Jamaica, some do attempt a show of bravado as they are being processed for reentry. But they often return with no material resources to give substance to the pretense. One such deportee is the subject of a fine Buju Banton morality tale, "Deportee (Things Change)."[18] A deportee is also the central character in a hilarious "roots play" produced by Ginger Knight, which featured Buju Banton's "Deportee" as theme song.

The DJ chastises the delinquent deportee who managed to acquire substantial wealth through criminal activities abroad. It is not so much the illicit nature of the income-generating activities of the deportee that is deplored; what is crucial is the deportee's profligacy. Like the biblical prodigal son, he squandered his ill-gotten gains in riotous living:

> Tings change
>
> Yu never send yu money come a yard.
>
> Yu wretch yu, yu spen di whole a it abroad
>
> Squander yu money
>
> Now yu living like dog
>
> ...
>
> Get deport
>
> Yu come dung [down] inna one pants

...

Remember how yu used to brag

Benz an Lexus a weh yu did have.

Furthermore, in violation of the common decency of sending remittances to less fortunate relatives "a yard," the deportee failed to maintain ties of kinship: "Not a letter, not a penny, not a fifty cents stamp." There is a mocking refrain throughout, "Back together again." That line, sampled from a celebratory pop song about reunited lovers, sardonically underscores the depth to which the deportee has fallen. He is now "back together again" with all those *back-a-yard* Jamaicans who failed in their bid to get a visa. He's right back where he started. In fact, he's probably worse off, "living like a dog." Retributive suffering becomes the just fate of the delinquent deportee.

The *Abeng* newsletter, which is published quarterly in a detention center in Stormville, New York, carried a 1998 feature article by Julian Cowell. The newsletter explores the issue of the international prisoner transfer treaty to which Jamaica is not a signatory and raises the problematic question of how the deportee is to be reintegrated into Jamaican society. The newsletter contests the "Deportee Bill" for its scapegoating of deportees: "It is the position of the Government of Jamaica that deported individuals are mainly responsible for the ballooning crime rate in Jamaica. This belief has led to legislation ('Deportee Bill') aimed at 'monitoring' deportees. The 'Deportee Bill' may well be found to be unconstitutional and furthermore may not have the desired impact on the twin problem of crime and violence." [21]

"Outernational" is thus not all benevolence and opportunities to "mek it" and to "live big." Some Caribbean migrants feel drawn to take risks outside the law—pushing drugs, for example. Within the law, migrants often have to work very hard at two or three jobs in order to make life, to have their fun, and, above all, to keep alive the hope of returning to their country of birth. This journey, if achieved outside a coffin, transforms the subject into a "returning resident"/"returnee." Jamaican historian and sociologist Winston James explores the somewhat macabre subject of the high cost of repatriating patriotic Jamaican corpses to a last resting place in the sun in the fascinating essay "Migration, Racism and Identity Formation: The Caribbean Experience in Britain."[20] The returnee who was so proudly, even aggressively "Jamaican" in all those years abroad, enduring cold temperatures and the chill of unlawful race discrimination, oftentimes clashes with the "stay-a-yard" Jamaican whose cultural practices are not always welcoming or familiar. The insidious stereotype of the "mad" Jamaican created by the alienating experience of migration to the United Kingdom, for example, evokes yet another border clash: on the threshold between alleged lunacy and sanity.[21]

One of the most controversial sites of contestation in Jamaican society, and which is fully documented in dancehall music, is the border clash between ghetto youth and state authority. This ongoing clash underscores the ideological continuities between contemporary dancehall music and traditional "conscious" reggae. Reggae came to international attention in the late 1960s and early 1970s as the music of a moment of social transformation nationally, regionally, and internationally. A major facet of that music was its protest-cum-revolutionary lyrical content and a profoundly ideological force within it was religious, specifically Rastafari.

The closure of those heady days of idealism was marked by the political demise in 1980 of Michael Manley's 1970s' experiment with socialism and the death of Bob Marley in 1981. Other markers include the coming to power of U.S. President Ronald Reagan and U.K. Prime Minister Margaret Thatcher. The movement for social transformation out of which Bob Marley, Peter Tosh, Bunny Wailer, Big Youth, and the Burning Spear spoke seemed to have been derailed. The Michael Manley "process" was defeated. The Jamaican Marxist Left appeared to have packed up voluntarily and gone home. The implosion of the Grenada Revolution, facilitating as it did the U.S. invasion, did not help the credit balance of socialism. The fall of the Berlin Wall and the rapid disappearance of the regimes of the world socialist camp in Eastern Europe were a serious challenge to the practical credibility of Marxism.

As the 1980s, that challenging decade of "market capitalism," wore on, cultures of both opposition and resistance had to adjust and were forced to "balance up and come again," as a triumphant sound system DJ once said dismissively to a faltering rival. We register here this "oppositional" versus "resistance" distinction not because we think it persuasive but because it has been given some credence in the literature on the Caribbean popular. A problematic discussion of the terms appears, for example, in Richard Burton's *Afro-Creole: Power, Opposition and Play in the Caribbean,* in which he attempts to explicate the distinction in his introduction: "I say 'resistance' in deference to standard usage, but, in fact, as readers will quickly discern, I draw an important distinction, derived from the work of Michel de Certeau . . . between 'resistance'—those forms of contestation of a given system that are conducted from *outside* that system, using weapons and concepts derived from a source or sources other than the system in question—and "opposition," by which term de Certeau designates those forms of contestation of a given system that are conducted from *within* that system, using weapons and concepts derived from the system itself."[22]

As is well known, in the early 1980s it became mortally dangerous in Jamaica to resist/oppose the system and to chant "truths and rights." The popular was pushed in another direction, giving rise to dancehall. For almost a decade, this new genre mainly expressed, reflected, even celebrated the carnal, the violent, and the slack. Mainly, but not wholly. And even within the culture of slackness could be seen the signs of a bare-faced, bare-bottomed subversion of the dominant social order.[23] The ever-increasing economic hardships and sociopolitical oppression drove the popular toward a head-on confrontation with the forces of repression. Importantly, Rastafari first survived and then achieved a kind of a triumph within the popular. Since the early 1990s it has come to dominate the chants of the "singers and players of instruments," especially the DJs, in the form of roots'n'culture/reality/consciousness music.[24]

The proponents of this revival are, in the main, astonishingly young, most in their early twenties; and the discourse is overwhelmingly masculine. These youths constitute a cluster, perhaps even a movement, the outriders of a dimly perceived reemerging radical Jamaican social movement. As Anthony B says in "One Thing":

> Every entertainer tek dem baptism
> Show to di world dat dem a Rastaman
> Anthony B, Little Devon have joined di gang
> Risto Benjie, Buju Banton
> Accept Selassie as the Almighty One.[25]

Anthony B adds more names to the list of baptized entertainers in a wide-ranging interview with David Scott: Capleton, Sizzla, Determine, Louie Culture, and Luciano.[26] It is primarily this righteous gang who now voice oppositional politics in Jamaica. And since Rastafari mines the King James version of the Bible for its most potent imagery, the call to arms for its converts is also a call to prayer. The revolution becomes eschatology, so to speak.

Accordingly, the social forces and individuals that are perceived by the DJs as the current enemies of the Jamaican people are imaged as long-ago entities Sodom and Gomorrah of the Old Testament and Babylon of the New. The Revelations of St. John the Divine assume a renewed character in the Jamaican popular, and this spiritually unimpeachable source, the Bible, inspires the incendiary element of the passionate discourse of the DJs that inflames immediate border clashes in today's Jamaica. The fire-and-brimstone rhetoric of this new generation of conscious DJs has quite a respectable pedigree, as is elaborated in chapter 6.

One of the most striking exponents of this genre is Anthony B, whose apocalyptic text "Fire Pon Rome" voices the new spirit.[27] That Rome and not Babylon is the primary city incinerated here speaks to the continuing power of the final book of the Bible in the Jamaican imagination. Rome is the city upon which the apostle heaped his terrible odium. The modern Italian city-state, home to the headquarters of the Roman Catholic Church, the Vatican, is never, on this African Jamaican cultural terrain, allowed to escape its ancient anathema. It matters not that the Ethiopian Orthodox Church, the formal religious home of many Rastafari, recognizes the Church of Rome as an ancient sister body within Christendom. Under the powerful influence of the book of Revelations, "Rome" in popular Rastafari discourse signifies institutionalized religion malfunctioning against the interests of poor people/ghetto people. It symbolizes Rastafari hatred of what is termed "church an' state philosophy."

Anthony B's compelling imprecations in "Fire Pon Rome" are part of a long-established oral tradition of warning in Jamaica.[28] The itinerant "warner," a terrifying street preacher, brings both a message of damnation and the promise of redemption if the evildoer forsakes the path of destruction. From the perspective of a child, Jamaican poet and literary critic Edward Baugh gives an emotive recollection of the shattering effect of one such warner-woman from his rural past:

> The morning shimmers in its bowl of blue crystal.
> Me, underneath my mother's bed.
> I delight in dust and dimness.
> Connoisseur of comics and the coolness of floorboards,
> I prolong my life's long morning.
>
> But the blue sky broke. The warner-woman.
> Bell-mouthed and biblical
> she trumpeted out of the hills,
> prophet of doom, prophet of God,
> breeze-blow and earthquake,
> tidal wave and flood.

I crouched. I cowered. I remembered Port Royal.

I could see the waters of East Harbour rise.

I saw them heave Caneside bridge. Dear God,

don't make me die, not now, not yet!

Well, the sky regained its blue composure.

Day wound slowly down to darkness.

Lunch-time came, then supper-time,

then dream-time and forgetting.

Haven't heard a warner-woman

these thirty-odd years.[29]

The warner-woman of Baugh's youth is not, in fact, silent but now speaks in the language and *riddim* of the dancehall. Thanks to the Scott interview, we know that Anthony B's remarkable "Fire Pon Rome" was composed in great passion and with visionary zeal for one of the most carnal and clash-oriented of shows, Sting. The DJ gives a contemplative account of the reasoning (in the Rastafari sense of the word) out of which the song was conceived and rapidly delivered in 1995:

Yu see Ah [I] was inna Bermuda—me, Luciano, Sizzla, Jesse Gender an di whole Exterminator Crew. An Sting was four days away. Wi miss di flight so wi didn't get fi do no rehearsal. So wi inna Antigua an wi a reason bout some vibes inna Jamaica an wi seh wa really a go on is dat there can be a better change inna di youth dem, but di youth will mek a change if dem see di elder dem mek di change. Because why di youth dem bruck [break] out is dat dem see di elder dem bruck out. Cause im a go look an see, who a lead wi, dem naa do notn [nothing], so it no mek sense we do something. So is dat deh vibe wi sidong [that vibe we sit down] an a reason bout. So me come home back now, two day before Sting an go dong pon di beach early a morning, an just hold a vibe. An is like a day before Sting it come to me, an mi tell it to Bobo . . . an Bobo seh is a good tune. It was backstage now at

Sting mi really finish it. Only di second verse mi have. An Bobo seh don't
bother go pon stage an DJ dat, yu know, because it no done. . . .[30]

To the best of our knowledge, "Fire Pon Rome" is the only work in the
Jamaican popular canon that invokes the names of the wealthy and the
politically powerful in such an explicit manner. In this regard, the calypso
always appeared more advanced than reggae; license, that ritual of rebellion, has been a major facet of annual carnival revelry in Trinidad and
Tobago. Those named by Anthony B are some of the leading owners of
capital—Azan, Matalon, and Butch Stewart; as well as the leaders of the
two main political parties—Prime Minister P. J. Patterson of the ruling
People's National Party and Edward Seaga, leader of the opposition
Jamaica Labour Party. Bruce Golding, former leader of the now-restruc-
tured New Democratic Movement, is also named. In another song, "Nah
Vote Again," Anthony B derisively dismisses all three parties as constituting a collective threat to the interests of the poor:

> Only ting wi get from election a death an problem
> Dem tell yu vote fi all di PNP
> We find out dat a *P*ains, *N*eeds an *P*overty
> Dem tell yu fi vote fi all di JLP
> Dat a *J*uicing di *L*ife of di ghetto *P*ikni
> NDM seh yu fi come vote fi D
> Yu no see a *N*ew *D*estruction for you an *M*e
> Dem a try bus [burst] Jamaicans inna three
> Mi a unite dem fi face God Almighty
> So wi nah vote again.[31]

Anthony B's disavowal of representational politics is reminiscent of
Louise Bennett's satirical critique of government programs and the elec-
toral process in poems such as "Census" and "Votin' Lis'," which subversively express working-class resistance to government interference in the

lives of the people. For example, in "Census," the speaker confesses her sabotaging of the reporting system on grounds of the nosiness of personified "Govament":

Jamaican:
But govament fas' ee mah? Lawd!
Me laugh soh tell me cry,
Me dis dun tell de census man
A whole tun-load o' lie.

Him walks een an sidung like is
Eena my yard him grow,
An yuh want to hear de femelia tings
De man did want fe know.

Him doan fine out one ting bout me,
For fe me y'eye soh dry,
Me stare right eena census face
An tell him ban o' lie![32]

English:
But isn't the Government nosey, my dear? Good Lord!
I laughed so hard I'm crying
I've just told the census officer
A ton of lies

He walked in and sat down as if
He grew up right here in this house
And you won't imagine all the personal details
This man wanted to know

He didn't learn a thing about me,

For I'm so brazen
I looked him straight in the eye
And told him a pack of lies

Similarly, in "Votin' Lis'" the speaker derides the aggressive verbal strategies of election campaigners and promises to undermine the voting system by defacing the ballot paper:

Jamaican:
Bans o' man all ovah islan',
Dis a-blista up dem t'roat
Dis a-chat till dem tongue leng out
An dah-beg me fe me vote.

Ah gwine meck dem tan deh beg me,
Ah gwine meck dem tan deh pine,
Ah gwine rag an haul an pull dem
So till ah meck up me mine.

Me doan know who me gwine vote fa,
For me doan jine no gang,
But what me cross out gawn like storm
An wat me lef kean wrong.[33]

English:
A lot of men all over the island
Are wasting a lot of breath
Chatting to the point of exhaustion
And begging me for my vote

I'm going to let them keep on begging
I'm going to let them keep on pining

I'm going to give them a run for their money
Until I make up my mind.

I don't know who I'm going to vote for,
For I haven't joined any of the gangs
But what I cross out will be completely erased
And what I leave can't be wrong.

It is instructive that Bennett uses the derogatory word "gang," with its criminal associations, to describe the political parties, thus foreshadowing Anthony B's righteous distancing of himself from the divide-and-rule politics of the three main parties.

Reporting on media responses to the radicalism of Anthony B's incisive lyrics, Scott asks: "But these talk-show hosts are saying that criticizing is one thing but that you are disrespectful to certain leaders. How do you respond to that?"[34] Anthony B's reply makes it seem, at first glance, as if he is in retreat from his militant posture. But, in fact, the cunning DJ undermines the very notion of disrespect by emphasizing the disingenuous nature of the question he asks in "Fire Pon Rome": "No, but you see, I am not disrespecting anybody. I wouldn't hold a mike and say, well Mr This is that and Mr That is this. I never spoke any disrespectful words. The first thing I say in the song is: 'This is my question to Issa and Mr Matalon/ How you come to own so much of black people's land?' Then, if any intelligent person, someone who has been to university and so on, comes up to you and asks how you come to own so much of black people's land, you simply have to give them an example: 'I own it as a result of buying it or doing this or that . . .'"[35]

Anthony B's innocuous-sounding question is a pointed critique of the post-slavery arrogation of the major resources of the colony (land, social territory, and finance) by Europeans, directly or though their control of the colonial state. Indeed, it is this problem of landlessness that occasioned the other core problem of post-emancipation African Jamaicans, namely wage slavery, which, admittedly, the DJ does not mention in this particular text. The issue of disrespecting "certain leaders" is thus an irrelevance. The DJ does not *diss* the financial powerbrokers and their political allies; he denounces them.

Anthony B's inspired text, "Fire Pon Rome," discloses the fundamental African Jamaican disaffection with the political system: "Outa politics poor people get dem beating." Politicians with their party politics, says the DJ, are central to the neocolonial problem, not its solution. Their "party politics" has not only failed to deliver any benefits to poor people, but partisan politics is itself a major structural means of exacerbating the deprivation of the poor. Anthony B elaborates this point in "Nah Vote Again," which, opening with a sample from the Ethiopians' 1969 hit "Everything Crash," underscores the intertextuality of the lyrics of the contemporary DJs and their reggae antecedents and demonstrates, as well, how little has changed, fundamentally, for the poor in the intervening years:

> Prologue:
>
> See it ya now
>
> Everything crash
>
> Wha gone bad a morning
>
> Can't come good a evening
>
> Dat's why
>
> Wi naa vote again
>
> All dem a enumerate
>
> Naa participate
>
> So wi naa vote again
>
> Only ting wi get from election
>
> A death an problem
>
> So wi naa vote again

The rejection of the methods of the constituted order is total, but violence is not advocated. There is in its place a confidence in the movement toward increasing understanding and unity among the people, in the face of which a Jah/God-ordained defeat of the forces of the ungodly enemy is certain. Thus, in "Swarm Me," Anthony B confidently asserts:

Dem know seh dat dem can't lose
Dis is di generation dem can't confuse
Dis is di generation dem can't use
Get di news.[36]

But it is not only the conscious youth who can no longer be manipulated by the political system. Even those whom Anthony B calls the "generation of vipers" renounce unswerving party affiliation for the immediate material benefits that are offered by those with the resources to buy loyalty, however fleeting. In the Scott interview Anthony B elaborates:

Dis is di unruly generation. Understand mi, man. Dis is a new generation now, dat Babylon can't go line up an seh you is a PNP an you is a Labourite. Dem youth no deh pan dat. Money! If a PNP a run [is handing out] money, im deh-deh [he's there]; if a Labourite a run money, im deh-deh. Yu see weh mi mean? So money is di controller of dem youth ya. Not no leader nor no man who dem *like*. Dem a youth ya no like *nobody*. Yu understand mi? Dis is di generation of vipers dat di Bible tell yu bout. So dis is di generation who will survive. . . . Dis is di generation who a deal wid survival. Dem naa follow no man an seh "yeah wi rate da man deh, wi a go tump [hit] a man inna im mouth fi dat man." No. Politician seh "go lik down da man deh," an dem go down and seh, "bwoy, a one millionaire dis! . . . Listen politician seh fi come lik yu down, gi mi a ting. . . ."[37]

The border clash between elitist politicians and the masses of the people invoked in "Fire Pon Rome" is also cross-generational. The youth are far more cynical about politics than their parents. In the words of Anthony B:

Well, see, first time now yu born as a lickle [little] youth, yu mother a PNP you is a PNP, yu father is Labourite you is a Labourite. Dat a dat. Yu just born an accept dat. But yu see now a youth born im a look a different ting fi imself. Im a look. Im a seh 'mi no have no time fi politics, mi want mi car, mi house, and mi want dat' an im a tink more of life dan just fi follow im parents. First time yu future did decide off a yu parents. Now a no so it go wid dem ya youth. If yu warn yu youth [child], it no mek no sense, yu a go lose im. Is wa im feel interested inna most.[38]

Another fundamental issue "sighted up" in "Fire pon Rome" is "mental slavery," the DJ thus echoing the words of Marcus Garvey and Bob Marley:

Burning fire
Black people don't get weary
Burning fire
Dem tek off di shackles an chains
Inna fire, hotter, hotter fire
An seh dem free wi
But wi still under mental slavery

Anthony B's allusion to Bob Marley's "Redemption Song" confirms the DJ's sense of lineage within a tradition of political radicalism to be found in reggae music and also in the African redemption philosophy of Marcus Garvey. His song "Marley Memories" is a personal tribute to Marley as well as a direct challenge to the state to honor Marley, de facto national hero, by putting his image on the thousand-dollar bill. Regretfully, the Jamaican elite missed an opportunity to heed Anthony B's call and conferred that honor instead on former Prime Minister Michael Manley:

Every national hero deh pon money
Paul Bogle, Sam Sharpe and Lady Nanny

Bustamante, Norman Manley an Marcus Garvey
Pon di thousand dollar bill wi waan see Bob Marley
Only Marcus alone do wa Bob Marley do fi wi.[39]

Like the ideological barrier between the politicians and the people, the border between capital and the masses is similarly aflame. The Jamaican labor market graphically illustrates capital's decreasing ability to manipulate the cheapened labor power of those in peripheral nation-states. In that instructive interview, Anthony B notes the entanglement of capital and politics in the continued oppression of the poor. In response to Scott's statement, "But, Anthony B, wa yu a seh is dat di politician dem no business wid poor people. Dem ongle business wid demself," the DJ concurs:

No, just dem an dem friend. Dem just come together, who inna di same circle, keep dem big party, an laugh about wa a gwaan. Dem is not about we. Di only time yu see dem dong inna di ghetto is now. Yu start see dem inna dis ya season now cause election a come. Yu never see dem weh day [in the recent past]. An none of dem no live ya. Dem live inna dis island and dis island, an dem carry di whole a dem money gone bank up deh so. An mi an yu have fi bank ya so. An when yu no bank inna fi yu country yu no put no investment inna yu country. If yu a tek your country money somewhe yu no di govament. Most a di govament money inna Cayman, it deh inna ya so an ya so. None of it no deh inna Jamaica a invest.[40]

Scott observes, in response to Anthony B's naming of the particular capitalists Azan, Matalon, Issa, and Butch Stewart, "These, in a sense are the old white merchant class. But there is in Jamaica today a class of black people who control significant wealth, for instance the financial sector."[41] But Anthony B does address Scott's point about the "ethnicity"/color of local capital and its agents in "Fire Pon Rome." It is clear in the song and from the DJ's answer in the interview that the issue is not just one of skin color; certainly not on its own. Oppression comes in many shades and guises. Hence the lines: "When yu look pon dem face/ A yu owna black man" [When you look on their face/ Is your own Black people.] This caveat would apply not just to the lowly enforcers of the regulations of the Metropolitan Parks and Markets (MPM) agency, which partly polices street trading, but also to many of the politicians denounced and especially to the prime minister himself. The focus of the text itself, as far as the named capitalists are concerned, is very specific indeed.

Here, also, Scott's question appears beside the point and somewhat misleading. The fact is that the financial sector, which he mentions, is—and was at the time the question was posed—in a massive crisis, prevented from being terminal only by the intervention of the government of Jamaica at the expense of the taxpayer. The effect of the massive "bailout" of the sector has been to commit over 70 percent of the national budget to the servicing of the national debt, major segments of which are rising at high rates of compound interest, and which now exceeds total gross domestic product. A number of the biggest failed financial institutions are precisely those run by the Black finance capitalists Scott would have had in mind.

Nor are the named capitalists best thought of as "the old white merchant class." They may have originated in this class, but their expanded stake in the Jamaican economy makes them much more than that. It is important to note that Butch Stewart is one of the biggest names in the old mode of merchandising and also in the modern hotel, tourism, and commercial air transport sectors. He is, as Anthony B says, the owner of Air Jamaica, which has been recapitalized and fully underwritten by Jamaican taxpayers. The Butch Stewart package is reinforced by ownership of a newspaper, the *Jamaica Observer*—handy for cross-subsidies on advertising.

Anthony B addresses the capitalists' control of land, which has made the Matalons, for example, major players in Jamaica's mass housing sector and in commercial property development. This is the burden of Anthony

B's barbed and accurate reference in "Fire Pon Rome" to the killing the Matalons have made out of the development of housing schemes in Portmore and beyond:

> Check out Greater Portmore, Braeton
>
> One room unu [you all] build a sell fi [is being sold for] one million
>
> Dem deh [those] studio house no worth a hundred gran.

Anthony B's reference to Azan, Matalon, and downtown Kingston highlights clashes taking place on still other Jamaican borders: those concerned with the policing of informal trading on the streets of downtown Kingston, which pits the immediate survival interest of the many poor against the merchant few who had, in any event, for years abandoned downtown for the New Kingston development, and for Miami and Toronto.

In "Fire Pon Rome" Anthony B also accuses his specified capitalists of running down parts of Kingston. The likely absence of working-class people from among the beneficiaries of the redevelopment of the downtown area is a related issue. Clashes between informal commercial importers (ICIs) and the combined force of the police and officers of the MPM were occurring downtown in 1995 when Anthony B's song was written and occur intermittently elsewhere in Jamaica. Incidentally, a Matalon was, at the time, head of the MPM. The ubiquitous ICI has become a potent symbol of the resilience of the working-class individual who, refusing to bow to the forces of economic oppression, struggles valiantly in small-scale trading to make a living. Some ICIs have had remarkable success, which has enabled them to move into middle-class residential areas, much to the distress of their snobbish neighbors who often disdain to acknowledge the presence of the "hurry-come-ups."

Buju Banton's anthemic "ICI," dedicated to up-and-coming entrepreneurs as well as more established figures in the field, is a masterly celebration of this social stratum and, within it, the market higgler.[42] In an act of resistance to state authority, Buju urges patronage of the working class ICI, whose economic activities have been declared illegal. Buying from the higgler, as distinct from the settled storeowner, thus becomes a subversive declaration of class war. The compelling argument Buju makes for keeping the higgler in business is this: she is valiantly struggling to make a living. So the DJ explicitly advises his audience against bypassing the street vendor or, worse, engaging in counterproductive activities such as sampling the higgler's food stock without making a purchase.

Turning from potential customers to the higglers themselves, the DJ exhorts the ICIs to keep jostling for space in the public sphere. Though born in poverty, many have managed to negotiate their way out of the concrete jungles of extreme deprivation. The successful higgler becomes emblematic of all disenfranchised people who desire upward social mobility and are prepared to work long and hard to achieve the leap. The DJ celebrates the ICI's refusal to idly sit at home waiting on remittances from abroad or for handouts from politicians at home. It is pride in self that motivates the undefeated higgler to engage in economic activities that are delegitimized by the state.

Claude McKay's jeremiad, "The Apple-Woman's Complaint," published in 1912 in his *Constab Ballads,* is an early-twentieth-century account of a long-running battle between mostly female itinerant vendors and the police. Like Buju's ICIs, the Apple-woman knows that she must depend on herself for her economic survival:

Jamaican:
While me deh walk 'long in de street,
Policeman's yawnin' on his beat;
An' dis de wud him chiefta'n say—
Me mus'n' car' me apple-tray

Ef me no wuk, me boun' fe tief;
S'pose dat will please de pólice chief!
De prison dem mus' be wan' full

Mek dem's 'pon we like ravin' bull.

. . .

Ah massa Jesus! In you' love
Jes' look do'n from you' t'rone above,
An' show me how a poo' weak gal
Can lib good life in dis ya wul'.[43]

English:
While I'm walking along in the street,
The policeman's yawning on his beat;
And this is the word his chieftain has issued—
I mustn't carry my apple-tray
If I don't work I'll be forced to steal
I suppose that will please the police chief!
They must want to fill up all the prisons,
That's why, like raving bulls, they're attacking.

. . .

Ah Dear Jesus! In your love
Just look down from your throne above,
And show me how a poor weak girl
Can live a good life in this world.

Nothing much has changed in nearly a century, it would seem.
Admittedly, arcades have been built to house the higglers and to encourage
their relocation from the streets. But the practical advantages of itinerant
vending are undeniable. In addition, the preferred location for many
higglers is not the somewhat isolated arcade but the storefront piazzas of
main street shops, in close proximity to potential clients. Shop owners
naturally resent this incursion on the prime public space in front of their
stores. Border clashes inevitably ensue. JLP Member of Parliament Pear-
nel Charles has proposed a novel solution to this seemingly intractable
problem of street vending: "'No solution to the problem that doesn't

involve the purchaser can solve it,' Charles told the *Observer*. 'What the government needs to do is declare certain areas in some sections of the city, non-business areas, and anyone, both buyer and seller, found transacting business in those areas should be charged. Make it a misdemeanour that will carry a fine.'"[44] Charles also points to the root of the conflict between higglers and shopkeepers: "The store owners created the dilemma by using the higglers at first to sell goods for them," he said. "After a while, the higglers realised that they could make more money for themselves and stopped selling for the merchants. That is why the store owners are now complaining."[45]

What we have demonstrated here is the multivalence of the concept "border clash" in Jamaican popular culture. The terrain is complex. What is certain is that popular culture—the low—does interrogate the high fearlessly. The youthful singers and players of instruments in Jamaica, whose voice is amplified by the global recorded music industry, are willing to risk the dangers of the border clash. They lay themselves on the line as spokespersons for the masses of the Jamaican people whose dissonant expressions of social malaise often are muffled in the official discourses of the nation.

TWO

Slackness Personified

Representations of Female Sexuality
in the Lyrics of Bob Marley
and Shabba Ranks

Bob "Tuff Gong" Marley and Rexton "Shabba Ranks" Gordon have both
achieved international superstar status as exponents of Jamaican popular
music and articulators of the cultural values embedded in roots reggae and
its dancehall flowering—Marley far more so and far more enduringly than
Gordon. Conventional wisdom in Jamaica, manifested in the popular
press and on numerous talk-show programs, valorizes Bob Marley's
politically charged reggae lyrics as the peak of "culture." Conversely,
Shabba Ranks's erotic dancehall *liriks* are stigmatized as base, misogynist
"slackness."[1] Beyond fundamentalist Jamaica, the reggae culture/dance-
hall slackness dialectic does have some currency, though the oppositional
ideology is not often so simplistically stated as in the following case.

Journalist Tom Willis, writing in London's *Sunday Times,* attempts to
establish an invidious comparison between loving Bob Marley and hateful
Shabba Ranks. The latter is described as "a black pop star who last year
asserted on TV that homosexuals 'deserve crucifixion,' and expressed

support for such peers as Buju Banton and Tippa I-Re, whose lyrics favour the quicker method of shooting."[2] I certainly do not endorse Ranks's heterophobia, nor can I condone Willis's canonization of Bob Marley as the nonthreatening, pacifist singer of "lilting love songs." Rewriting history in an article entitled "Ragga to Riches," Willis proceeds to elaborate his facile distinction between the love lyrics of his one-dimensional Bob Marley and the uniformly violent lyrics of all of the performers of contemporary ragga: "Not that ragga, born in the violent dance halls of mid-1980's Kingston, bears much relation to Marley's lilting love-songs of the decade before. Rather than sing, the vocalists 'toast' in high-speed verse; patois lyrics have often celebrated misogyny, homophobia, gangsterdom and guns."[3]

But what of Marley's own songs of class war? Willis's generalization engenders a series of clear-cut oppositions: hate ragga versus Bob Marley's love songs; 1980's violence versus 1970's peace (presumably); toasting versus singing; "lilting" versus "high-speed"; (English) love songs versus patois lyrics—the contrast with English is implied in Willis's pointed reference to "patois" lyrics; hateful "misogyny, homophobia, gangsterdom and guns" versus unqualified love, pure and simple.

A decade later, Peter Thatchell, spokesperson for the UK gay rights group OutRage, echoes Willis's all too easy distinction between an unequivocally peaceful Bob Marley and the entire lot of unrepentantly combative DJs. Thatchell, who is currently leading a militant campaign to ban Jamaican DJs from performing in the UK anti-gay lyrics that are perceived to incite violence, is quoted in a *Gleaner* article: "We did it to Guns and Roses and to Marky Mark in the 90s and now we are saying to these dancehall artistes and producers if they refuse to desist [*sic*] inciting violence against lesbians and gays they will suffer the consequences. Everytime [*sic*] a concert is announced our aim will be to get it cancelled until these artists comply. . . . We want to drive homophobia out of dancehall music and to make life safe for lesbian and gay people. It's wrong that anyone should incite violence against another human being. We'd like to see Jamaican music reclaimed for Bob Marley's spirit of peace and brotherhood."[4]

As I argue in *Noises in the Blood,* the relatively few love songs composed and performed by Marley are an essential part of the larger corpus of revolutionary political texts. They demonstrate the versatility of this exceptional musician and, more broadly, confirm the multifacetedness of the roots reggae genre: not just social protest but also songs of seduction. But Willis's misrepresentation of Bob Marley as an exclusively lovey-dovey lyricist diminishes the range and resonance of the revolutionary work of the incendiary "Tuff Gong" Rastaman whose songs of emancipation from mental slavery are a powerful, denunciatory chant against oppressive state power in all its various guises.[5]

Willis's oversimplification aside, there is a decided continuity of subversive values between reggae "culture" and ragga "slackness." For example, Bob Marley's provocative line, "I want to disturb my neighbour," from the song "Bad Card" on the *Uprising* album, can be heard as a disquieting anthem for dancehall culture: the politics of noise.[6] Music is not mere entertainment but ideological weaponry, disturbing the peace. Furthermore, uneasy peace cannot be sustained, in the long term, at the expense of social justice. In the words of Peter Tosh:

> Everyone is crying out for peace, yes
> None is crying out for justice
> I don't want no peace
> I need equal rights and justice.[7]

Bob Marley's dis/concerting noise is not just literal, megawattage night music that disturbs a neighbor's sleep. Noise engenders a politics of disturbance and disruption, a destabilization of the moral majority's complacent rhythms of social decorum:

> You a go tired fi see mi face

Can't get mi out of the race

Oh man you said I'm in your place

And then you draw bad card

A make you draw bad card

. . .

I want to disturb my neighbour

Cause I'm feeling so right

I want to turn up my disco

Blow them to full watts tonight

Inna rub-a-dub style.[8]

"Rub-à-dub style," the noisy idiom of Bob Marley's explosive class politics, is also the erotic body language of the DJs. In the "rub-a-dub" aesthetics of the dancehall, carnality and social protest converge. But the carnality of the contemporary dancehall DJs often masks the political content of the discourse. Their distinctive rhythms of resistance, to cite Bob Marley's "One Drop," are not usually acknowledged as political. Furthermore, there is that new generation of "conscious" dancehall DJs who, disdaining the disguises of their "slackness" counterparts, have reclaimed a political militancy, a fight for truths and rights, that aligns them with the earlier reggae history of social protest.

But even that politically conscious reggae tradition is much more textured than is often acknowledged. The erotic was contained in the protest and often disrupted the simple logic of ascetic cultural warfare. This seductive tension between the erotic and the political continues to energize the dancehall, rub-a-dub style. Acknowledgment of this carnal element in "conscious" reggae makes it possible to hear the continuities in the work of the contemporary "slackness" DJs and that of their forebears. Bob Marley's "Kinky Reggae" exemplifies this slack/sensual streak in his work. Somewhat like Beenie Man's "real ghetto gyal" who gives the "wickedest slam," Marley's downtown "Miss Brown" offers exciting, kinky possibilities.[9] But Marley is decidedly ambivalent about his desire for Miss Brown's sugary boogawooga. Like the stereotypical uptown man to whom Beenie Man sings the praises of the real ghetto gyal, Marley confesses that his attraction to downtown Miss Brown is of the fleet-footed "hit and run" variety:

> I went downtown
> I saw Miss Brown
> She had brown sugar
> All over her boogawooga
> I think I might join the fun
> But I had to hit and run
> See I just can't settle down
> In a kinky part of town[10]

Issues of class aside, many middle-aged reggae fans, romanticizing their long-forgotten, lustful youth, selectively remember the good old boogawooga days. The complex fusion of the political and the erotic that has always characterized reggae music is reduced to simple sentimentality. A classic example of this revisionist impulse is Beresford Hammond's seductive hit song "Rock Away," a nostalgic anthem for that seemingly lost culture of "rent-a-tile" romance.[11] Hammond disarmingly encodes the very antagonisms of Willis's simplistic reading of Marley versus the contemporary DJs: in the heyday of the reggae singers and the old-style DJs, "love used to reign."[12] By contrast, the modern dancehall is a site of war: "now there's hardly any safe place left to go/ Someone's bound to come and try to spoil the show, oh oh."[13] Hammond elaborates:

> Oh yeah
> Oh I miss those days yeah
> I miss those days yeah
> Remember the songs used to make you rock away
> Those were the days when love used to reign, hey
> We danced all night to the songs they played

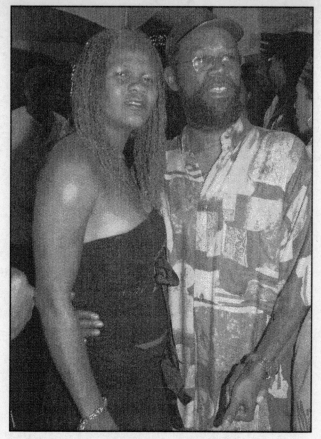

Lady Saw and Beres Hammond enjoying themselves at the Puma/VP
Jamaican Celebration at the Terra Nova Hotel in December 2003.
Photo: Ian Allen.

Weekend come again, do it just the same, hey

Now I feel it to my heart

Being such a golden time had to part, yes[14]

Hammond gives a lyrical salute to the old school greats, the honor roll
including not just reggae/lovers rock singers and the foundation DJs but
also R&B/soul crooners:

> Hail John Holt, Alton Ellis, Delroy Wilson,
> Dennis Brown, hey, hey
> Big Youth, Josey Wales,
> Daddy Roy would wake the town, yeah
> And you hold your woman real close
> When Smokey starts to sing
> Temptations, Marvin Gaye, Spinners all the way
> Aretha Franklin, Patti LaBelle
> Used to make me drift away
> Play, Stevie, play
> Sam Cooke any day, yeah[15]

From Hammond's perspective, there is little of value in the contemporary dancehall scene. So it must be erased:

> Right now we need a brand new start
> People everywhere need more music from the heart
> And there remains such a place that I can go
> Will someone tell me, tell me, I want to know
> Remember the songs used to make you rock away
> Those were the days when love used to reign, hey[16]

Love versus war; lovers rock/R&B versus today's dancehall; "music from the heart" versus *riddims* from the gut and the pelvis, it would seem. But Hammond selectively forgets that *fight used to bruck at dance* in those good old days. Love did not always reign. Human nature really has not changed in the intervening years. Sexual jealousy, for example, generated conflicts. The weapons of choice then were usually the intimate ratchet knife and broken beer bottle, not today's impersonal gun. The "safe place" of the past that Hammond now idealizes is likely to have been far more troublesome than his lyrical re-presentation of it. Furthermore, in the contemporary dancehall, all of the music from Hammond's "golden time" continues to be played alongside the current "big tunes." Hammond himself is a perennial hit.

Like Hammond, Barbara Gloudon, veteran journalist and a solid pillar of Jamaican society, romanticizing the good old days of "clean" reggae, lamented the "dirt" of current dancehall music at a 2002 symposium convened at the University of the West, Mona in honor of Clement "Sir Coxsone" Dodd: "I would like to see a Jamaica whe[re] cleanliness come back to it: emotional, physical cleanliness. A dutty country gwine produce dutty people weh gwine produce dutty music weh only dutty people want." [A dirty country is going to produce dirty people who are going to produce dirty music that only dirty people would want.] Though I understand Mrs Gloudon's passion for cleanliness, I could not resist the temptation immediately to challenge her seemingly indiscriminate dismissal of all of the contemporary creators of Jamaican popular music—and their enthusiastic fans—as "nasty nayga."[17]

In this sound clash between reggae and dancehall, Ninjaman's "Test the High Power," for example, illustrates the supposedly paradoxical way in which a lover's rock tune can be drawn by a canny selector, even in response to gun lyrics, in order to "kill" another sound system.[18] Ninjaman here recalls how he once brandished a Dennis Brown song, "Love and hate could never be friends," to remarkable effect: The crowd goes wild; bad men "clean" their guns; policemen return fire and, in the process, shoot ackees off a tree, kill a pigeon and set off a chain reaction as the dead bird falls on the head of a man in the dance, almost killing a Rastaman. Ninjaman's tall tale is an excellent example of the humorous quality of much of the banter in the supposedly "violent" arena of the sound clash. Indeed, this element of nonsensical verbal play is characteristic of Jamaican word games and illustrates the continuities between contemporary dancehall discourse and its more respectable antecedents.

The instinct of some older people to strictly segregate popular music of different historical periods into mutually exclusive categories is not shared by many youths whose taste in music is far more eclectic than their elders', as illustrated in the following anecdote. A colleague at the University of the West Indies, a historian, once told me that he couldn't find some of his classic reggae CDs and kept wondering where they could be; he didn't remember lending them out. He was most surprised to discover that his eleven-year-old son had appropriated them. But this is a child who had grown up on IRIE FM's regular feature, "Reggae for Kids," and who eagerly looked forward to the segment each weekday morning. So it should not have surprised his father that the child was now exploring this genre on his own. Misreading both reggae and dancehall, shortsighted historians of Jamaican popular music often fail to recognize continuities across seemingly fixed generic boundaries, routinely emphasizing, instead, absolute differences of tone, tempo, and temper.

There are obvious points of intersection between old school reggae and dancehall. For example, Bob Marley's incendiary, confrontational lyrics of class war and Shabba Ranks's explicit, hard-core celebration of X-rated sexuality share a common concern with destabilizing the social space of the respectable middle class. The lyrics of both artists articulate an antiestablishment class politics and a gender politics—admittedly, in crucially different ways. The "equal rights and justice" of Marley and Tosh are conceived in overtly political and socioeconomic terms. Shabba's equal rights are largely sexual, a masculinist/feminist assertion of egalitarian (sexual) relations between men and women. In the spirit of benevolent patriarchy, Shabba exhorts women to control the "commodification" of their body and ensure that men value them appropriately. This constitutes a radical politics and economics of the sexual body. Here I acknowledge Shabba Ranks's *consciously* articulated sexual politics, though I do concede an obvious rhetorical difference between the language of Shabba's performance and the language of my analysis.

This issue of language is complicated by sociocultural prejudices in Jamaica that would question both Shabba's ability to conceptualize and the capacity of the Jamaican language adequately to express abstract concepts such as I read in his lyrics. The problem of authorial "intention" is not, of course, peculiar to oral performance contexts. But in neocolonial Jamaica, more skeptical, color/class-coded readings than mine would challenge any assumption of Shabba's awareness of the full ideological implications of his own lyrics. For example, a female university student who read a draft of this chapter commented, with much condescension: "Poor Shabba no know seh a all dem tings deh im a seh" [Poor Shabba doesn't know that it's all of that he's saying].

But Shabba Ranks is, indeed, a perceptive analyst of the contentious social issues highlighted in his lyrics. In some of his songs he explicitly offers a self-critical analysis of the discourses in which he is implicated. For example, in "Back and Belly Rat" he militantly denounces the local print media for the bad press he receives, noting that it is his mastery of slackness lyrics, which the girls want, that has made his career. If there was no market for the product he could not succeed.[19] Furthermore, in "Just Reality," Shabba demonstrates his knowledge of Black history, citing Malcolm X, Martin Luther King, Marcus Garvey, Bob Marley and the contemporary Jamaican poet and public intellectual, Mutabaruka, as prime signifiers. Somewhat ironically, the DJ asserts that even Marley's liberation lyrics are not enough to truly emancipate some conniving Black people from divide-and-rule politics. Shabba contemptuously dismisses the invective of those who, averse to his sexual politics, begrudge his success. Defining an African genesis for his particular brand of "roots culture an reality," the DJ seems to be claiming a space for "slackness" as a legitimate politics that is broadly defined as synonymous with "reality."

In Jamaican popular culture, sexuality, like language, is a domain in which a political struggle for the control of social space is articulated. The body of woman, in particular, is the site of an ongoing struggle over high culture and low, respectability and riot, propriety and vulgarity. Woman embodies the slackness/culture dialectic in Jamaican popular culture. Somewhat paradoxically, Bob Marley's sexual politics is much more conservative than Shabba Ranks's apparently exploitative "sexism," with its ample references to the female body. Marley's gender politics, rooted in a sexually conservative Rastafari ideology, articulates a rather repressive vision of female sexuality. Marginalized Rastafari, as much as respectable, mainstream middle-class culture, does seek to extend its sexist control over the body of woman.

In Rastafari sexual politics, transgressive woman, synonymous with Babylon as whore, becomes an alluring entrapper, seducing the Rastaman from the path of righteousness. The biblical image of woman as fallen Eve/Babylonian whore defines contemporary gender relations that are founded on the essential frailty of both male and female flesh. The female is duplicitly represented as both deceiving and vulnerable to deception. For example, in Marley's "Waiting in Vain," from the *Exodus* album, the lover's ardent supplication modulates into definite reproof. The song confirms the ambivalent representation of woman—and male desire—in Bob Marley's lyrics and, more broadly, in Rastafari. Here are echoes of the "hit and run" doublespeak of "Kinky Reggae." The dilatory woman, with a long line of lovers in attendance, seems, in the man's view, to be functioning somewhat like a whore. The all-too-willing Rastaman is forced to patiently wait to negotiate a space for himself, however much he may not want to wait in vain.

The tension between the wanting and the waiting defines the pathos of this song:

I doan wanna wait in vain for your love

From the very first time

I blessed my eyes on you girl

My heart says follow through

But I know now that I'm way down on your line

But the waiting feel is fine

So don't treat me like a puppet on a string

Cause I know how to do my thing

Don't talk to me as if you think I'm dumb

I wanna know when you gonna come

See, I doan wanna wait in vain for your love.[20]

"Pimper's Paradise," from the *Uprising* album, is the classic example in Bob Marley's repertoire of that ambiguous Rastafari response to "fallen woman" as temptress: both attraction and repulsion, condemnation and empathy. It is the woman who allegedly initiates the fall, which the man himself thoroughly enjoys. Nevertheless, it is the woman who is scapegoated. "Pimper's Paradise" opens with the Rastaman's indictment of the fashion-conscious, pleasure-seeking, drug-addicted woman:

> She loves to party
> Have a good time
> She looks so hearty
> Feeling fine
> She loves to screw,
> Sometime shifting coke
> She'll be laughing
> When there ain't no joke
> A pimper's paradise
> That's all she was now.
> . . .
> She loves to model
> Up in the latest fashion
> She's in the scramble
> And she moves with passion
> She's getting high
> Trying to fly the sky, eh!
> Now she is bluesing
> When there ain't no blues.[21]

But the enigmatic line "Every need got an ego to feed"[22] does suggest empathy, however muted, for the woman who has perverted natural desire into self-destructive obsession. The reference to paradise subtly connotes Eve's fall from innocence, seduced by Satan, the original great pretender.

The song moves toward a clear statement of sympathy: "I'm sorry for the victim now."[23] The singer then addresses the woman directly, abandoning the initial, dismissive "throw-word" stance:

> Pimper's paradise
> Don't lose track
> Don't lose track of yourself, oh no!
> Pimper's paradise
> Don't be just a stock,
> A stock on the shelf
> Stock on the shelf[24]

The woman becomes more than exploited commodity; she is challenged to reclaim her humanity.

The ambiguous response to promiscuous woman in Marley's lyrics, as exemplified in "Pimper's Paradise," contrasts markedly with the uninhibited celebration of female sexuality in dancehall culture. In the words of Shabba Ranks:

> Jamaican:
> Who seh dat woman can done?
> Tell dem seh di woman don't come to done.
> One jook, one wash
> An den yu turn it down again
> Open yu foot
> A next man welcome.[25]

> English:
> Who says that woman can be exhausted?
> Tell them that
> Women don't come to be (un)done
> One poke, one wash

And then you turn it down again

Open your foot

Another man is welcome.

In Jamaican, "done" refers to both completion of an action and depletion of resources. This line from Shabba Ranks's song "Ca'an Dun" is primarily an allusion to the proverbial sexual plenitude of woman, in contrast to man's finitude. Admittedly, a less-flattering reference to woman is encoded here. "Woman can't done" also can be interpreted to mean that there is an inexhaustible supply of commodified women available for male consumption. In addition, the reference to washing and turning down again, as of dinnerware, suggests the promiscuous use-value of woman as vessel.

But the gender politics of the dancehall that is often dismissed by outsiders as simply misogynist can be read in a radically different way as a glorious celebration of full-bodied female sexuality, particularly the sub-stantial structure of the Black working-class woman whose body image is rarely validated in the middle-class Jamaican media, where eurocentric norms of delicate female face and figure are privileged. The recurring references in the DJs' lyrics to fleshy female body parts and oscillatory functions do not simply signify a clear-cut devaluation of female sexuality; rather, they signal the reclamation of active, adult female sexuality from the entrapping passivity of sexless Victorian virtue.

For example, in "Gone Up," from the *As Raw as Ever* 1991 CD, Shabba, playing on the proverbial association between food and sex in Caribbean culture, notes that the price of a number of commodities is going up: "Crotches! Sausage! Everything is going up. Bully beef, rice."[26] To a chorus of affirmative female voices, he asks women a rather pointed question and proceeds to give advice on negotiating a mutually beneficial sexual contract:

Jamaican:

Woman, wa unu a do fi unu lovin?

(Wi a raise it to)

Before yu let off di work

Yu fi defend some dollars first

Mek a man know seh

Ten dollar can't buy French cut

...

No mek no man work yu out

Body line, old truck.[27]

English:

Women, what are you going to do

About your loving?

(We are raising [the price of] it, too)

Before you have sex

You must make sure to negotiate first

Let the man know that

Ten dollars can't buy French cut [lingerie]

Don't let the man work over

Your body [as if it's an] old truck.

Shabba makes it clear that he is not advocating prostitution. The complicated relationships between men and women cannot be reduced to purely economic terms of exchange. He asserts that a man must assume a measure of social and economic responsibility for his sexual partner; it is, ultimately, a moral issue:

Jamaican:

Is not a matter a fact seh dat unu a sell it.

But some man seh dat dem want it.

As dem get it, dem run gone lef it.

No mek no man run gone lef it

An yu no get profit

Everything a raise, so weh unu a do?

Unu naa raise di price a unu pum-pum to?[28]

English:

It's not that you're actually selling it.

But some men say that they want it.

As soon as they get it, they run away and leave it.

Don't let the man run away and leave it

And you don't profit

Everything is going up so what are you going to do?

Aren't you going to raise the price of your pussy too?

Indeed, Shabba challenges the stereotype of the robotic, domesticated female who is too timid to question the unequal exchange of services and resources in her household:

Jamaican:

Have some woman gwaan like

dem no worth

Hitch up inna house like a house robot

House fi clean, dem clean dat up

An clothes fi wash, dem wash dat up

An dollars a run an dem naa get enough[29]

English:

There are some women who behave as if they have no worth

Confined to the house as though they are house robots

House to be cleaned, they clean it

Clothes to be washed, they wash them

Dollars are flowing and they don't get enough

Shabba scathingly indicts irresponsible men who, instead of spending money to support their household, would rather waste their resources carousing with their male cronies:

> Jamaican:
> Now yu have some man no want do no spending
> Dem uda do di spending pon dem bredrin
> An naa buy dem darling a icymint[30]

> English:
> Now there are some men who don't want to spend
> They would rather spend all their money on their male friends
> And wouldn't buy even an icymint for their darling

An icymint is one of the cheapest sweets on the market. The depth of the delinquent man's failure is thus measured in very common currency.

The DJ's compassion for female house robots and his equal contempt for sexist males who are stingy in domestic matters echo the critique of gender relations that Jamaican folklorist and poet Louise Bennett offers in her dramatic monologue "Oman Equality":

> Jamaican:
> Nuff oman deh pon a seh dat dem a seek liberation from man-dominance, counta how some man got a way fi chat bout seh "Woman's place is in the home," an a demands seh dat oman tan a yard so wash an cook an clean all day long, an teck any lickle money pittance what de husband waan fling pon dem a week time, an meck it stretch fi provide food an clothes an shelter, meanwhile de husban-dem a drink an gamble as dem like.[31]

> English:
> A lot of women are insistently seeking liberation from the dominance of men who advocate that a woman's place is in the home. These men demand that the woman stay at home, washing and cooking and cleaning all day long.

Then, at the end of the week, she is forced to take whatever pittance the husband throws her way. She has to make do with the little she gets, stretching it to cover the cost of food, clothing and shelter, while he's drinking and gambling as he pleases.

Bennett is not a writer whom one would readily identify with the "slackness" of dancehall culture, though I do argue that her choice of Jamaican as the preferred language of verbal creativity does align her to an outlaw tradition of resistance to eurocentric, uppercase High Culture. Contesting this argument, Ian Boyne declares: "There will be those who will seek to validate their vulgarity and cultural perversion by appealing to Miss Lou, noting the resistance she received from 'society people' when she started with the dialect. But don't involve Miss Lou inna unno [in your] nastiness. Everyone who knows her knows she hated profanity with a passion. Lady Saw is no modern-day Miss Lou! Vulgarity and the 'skin out, bruk out' thing is not our 'culture.' It is imported from abroad."[32] But there are, indeed, rare hints of sexual slackness in Louise Bennett's repertoire. Mervyn Morris, in his teaching notes to her poem "Registration," uncovers the sexual double-entendre in the following lines:

Jamaican:
Lawd-amassi, me feel happy
For me glad fi see at las
Oman dah meck up dem mine fi
Serve back man dem sour sauce![33]

English:
Lord have mercy, I feel happy
For I'm glad to see that at last
Women have made up their minds
To serve men their own sour sauce

Morris notes that "sauce here suggests semen; it is implied that women have decided to do to men what, sexually, men have done to them."[34]

Shabba, underscoring the fundamental necessity of sweet and sour sauce—both sex and food—urges men to assume economic responsibility for the eating that they do:

Jamaican:

Just like how a man can't live without flour

Or how a man can't live without rice

A so a man cannot live without wife

Yu have di uman

Spend nuff pon her right[35]

English:

Just as a man can't live without flour

Or a man can't live without rice

In the same way, a man can't live without a wife

If you have a woman

Spend a lot on her, [as is only] right

Although some women will decidedly object to the DJ's equating of rice/flour/wife, what is paramount here is Shabba's undermining of the popular middle-class Jamaican stereotype of the irresponsible working-class "baby-father," who assumes neither social nor economic responsibility for his woman and offspring.

Similarly, in "Woman Tangle," Shabba warns baby fathers against delinquency:

Jamaican:

If a woman out deh

Ha a baby fi yu

Bwoy, hold yu baby
An no mek it raffle.[36]

English:
If a woman out there
Gives birth to your baby
Man, hold on to your baby
Don't let it to have to be raffled.

The metaphor of the raffle cleverly suggests the dicey nature of the domestic affairs of irresponsible men. The image also alludes to the fact that unwanted children, who have lost the game of chance that gave them birth, often are placed in risky circumstances. For example, state-run children's homes in Jamaica are increasingly coming under scrutiny as sites of potential exploitation of helpless minors.[37]

In "Park Yu Benz" Shabba, asserting that material possessions are not enough to seduce women, mockingly challenges impotent men who have only money to offer women. Women want sexual satisfaction as much as material security: "Better park yu Benz an park yu BM/ If yu can't work yu uman she naa stay den"[38] [You'd better park your Benz and park your BMW/ If you can't satisfy your woman sexually she won't stay then.] In the following lines, Shabba liberally concedes the woman's freedom to have at least two male partners—one for "work" [sex] and one for "spend" [money]. Somewhat ironically, since "work" is a metaphor for sex in Jamaican, the man is spent, however the woman takes it. Shabba thus undermines the unequal gender politics that allows men the presumed right to have numerous sexual partners and, simultaneously, attempts to curtail women:

Jamaican:
One man want have twenty gyal-friend
An him woman must keep ongle one man-friend.
If a woman she have two man-friend,

One fi work, one fi spend

Dat is no problem.

Di one weh a spend, him have a problem.

Di one weh can work, him have all argument.

One man have forty-five girl friend

Through di neighbourhood him is a legend.

A gyal she go keep five man-friend

Is no prestige no more, she is ongle a spweng.[39]

English:

One man wants to have twenty girlfriends

And his woman must have only one sexual partner.

If a woman has two male friends,

One for sex, one for money

That's not a problem.

The one spending money, he has a problem.

The one who is good in bed, he has all the say.

One man has forty-five girlfriends

Throughout the neighborhood he is a legend.

A girl keeps five male friends

There's no more prestige, she's only a slut.

"Flesh Axe" similarly asserts the women's desire for both money and sex. Using agricultural, legal, and mechanical imagery, Shabba compares the body of woman to valuable property—land that must be cleared, seeded, and watered. Again, some women will object to the "commodifying" analogy. But in an agricultural economy that has long deprived small farmers of access to arable land, this earthy metaphor signifies the high value that is placed on the fertile body of woman. Furthermore, the vigorous metaphor of chopping the body land, which may sound disturbingly sadomasochistic to some ears, is a vivid sexual metaphor celebrating the efficiency of the phallic axe as it clears the ground for the planting of the seed. The hard labor of fieldwork is transmuted into pleasurable sexual work:

Jamaican:

Flesh axe

Di land pon di body fi chop

Is like money an woman sign a contract

If yu a deal wid a woman fi a natural fact

Is not seh dat she a sell her body

Fi run it hot

But every woman need mega cash

Fi buy pretty shoes an pretty frock

Woman love model an dem love fi look hot

She can't go pon di road a look like job lot

Every woman a go call her riff-raff

Look like a old car mash up an crash[40]

English:

Flesh axe

The body-land must be cleared

It's as though money and woman have signed a contract

If you're really going to deal with a woman

It's not that she's actually selling her body

And it's running at high speed

But every woman needs big bucks

To buy pretty shoes and pretty dresses

Women love to show off and they love to look hot

She can't go out on the road looking like job lot goods

Every woman is going to call her riff-raff

Looking like an old car all smashed and crashed

"Muscle Grip," from the *X-Tra Naked* CD, makes it clear that women are not merely passive, desired objects. Their active interest in their own sexual satisfaction requires a high degree of physical fitness to do the work. The recurring use of the word "work" for sex clearly denotes the stamina that is required. The skillful, acrobatic dancing that women do in serious foreplay—bending over backward and touching the ground, for example—is not for the physically unfit. The emphasis on the mobility of the woman's bottom, the seat of pleasure, is particularly pronounced. The wearing of the "batty-rider" emphasizes the woman's gross assets.[41] In a witty essay "Venus Envy," first published in the *Village Voice,* cultural critic Lisa Jones revives the early-nineteenth-century "Hottentot Venus" as the alluring progenitor of contemporary (Euro-American) images of desirable Black female sexuality: "A veritable butt revolution has swept America in the last two decades—brought to you by black music, designer jeans, and MTV. (Once you've seen Janet Jackson gyrate to 'Black Cat,' can you really go back to Twiggy?)"[42] The same question, asked in Jamaica: "Once you've seen the perennial dancehall queen Carlene 'skin out' to any dancehall tune, can you really go back to Miss Jamaica?"

In a highly competitive marketplace women have to ensure that they have pull. Undermining the eurocentric, chivalric romance of woman as delicate flower, Shabba recommends a robust muscularity that grips and holds the woman's sexual partner, literally. The pun on "hold" is multilayered. The English "hold" loses its final consonant in Jamaican, becoming "hole," as both noun and verb[43]:

Jamaican:

Woman, yu pretty laka flowers

Dat alone naa go do

Although yu pretty so, man still a lef yu

Yu look good, from a look good point of view

Although yu look good, woman dem look good to

If yu can't hold yu man, a gyal a tek im from yu

Have di grip, have di muscle, him have fi come back to yu[44]

English:

Woman, even if you're as pretty as a flower

That alone won't be enough
Although you're that pretty, the man will still leave you
You may look good, from a purely superficial point of view
Although you do look good, other women look good too
If you can't hold on to your man
Another woman will take him from you
Have the grip, have the muscle tone
He'll have to come back to you.

The DJ's pragmatism in matters of sexual politics is firmly rooted in Jamaican peasant values. A number of Jamaican proverbs suggest the clear correlation of love, sex, and money in folk culture:

1. When money done, love done.
2. Man can't marry if him don't have cashew.
3. When man have coco-head[45] in a barrel, him can go pick wife.
4. When pocket full, and bankra[46] full, woman laugh.
5. Cutacoo[47] full, woman laugh.
6. Woman and wood, and woman and water, and woman and money never quarrel.[48]
7. You must find a place to put your head before you find a hole to put your hood.

Comparative analysis of the representation of female sexuality in the lyrics of Bob Marley and Shabba Ranks reveals changes in Jamaican cultural politics as the society evolves from a rural, peasant-based agricultural economy to an urban, wage-earning economy. Old-fashioned peasant values of relatively settled domestic order on small landholdings give way to more modern notions of commodified exchange of goods and services in relatively unstable urban settlements. Sexual relations between men and women often reflect prevailing socioeconomic conditions. It is not only sexual relations that are now commercialized in the urban setting. For example, informal, communal child-care systems in rural areas give way to the organized business of the urban day-care industry.

Bob Marley's somewhat chauvinist Rastafari lyrics issue, in part, from the conservative, biblically grounded peasant values of his rural origins. The secular economics of Shabba Ranks's much more egalitarian gender politics may be read as an urban updating of the proverbial wisdom of Jamaican folk culture. It is not only woman that is inexhaustible; Jamaican popular culture keeps on renewing itself, transforming norms of sexual decorum to suit the material conditions of the changing times.

THREE

Lady Saw Cuts Loose
Female Fertility Rituals in the Dancehall

Iyalode Oshun. Goddess of the River. Daughter of
Promise. Mother of the Sweet Waters.
It is from your throbbing Womb that the rhythm of Music
springs. It is from your bouncing Breasts that Dance is born.[1]

—Luisah Teish, "Daughter of Promise"

The flamboyantly exhibitionist DJ Lady Saw epitomizes the sexual liberation of many African Jamaican working-class women from airy-fairy
Judaeo-Christian definitions of appropriate female behavior. In a decisive
act of feminist emancipation, Lady Saw cuts loose from the burdens of
moral guardianship. She embodies the erotic. But one viewer's erotica is
another's pornography. So Lady Saw is usually censured for being far too
loose—or "slack," in the Jamaican vernacular. Or worse, is dismissed as a
mere victim of patriarchy, robbed of all agency. Marian Hall's spectacular
performance of the role of "Lady Saw" is not often acknowledged as a
calculated decision by the actress to make the best of the opportunity to
earn a good living in the theater of the dancehall.

For example, American anthropologist Obiagele Lake indicts Lady Saw in a chapter on "Misogyny in Caribbean Music": "Given Jamaica's patriarchal climate, one would expect sexist lyrics emanating from men. Unfortunately, women who have internalized sexist norms add to these negative images. Lady Saw is one such songstress who plays herself and, by association, all other women. 'Stab Up (sic) the Meat' is the most graphic example."[2] The title of this raunchy song is, in fact, "Stab Out Mi Meat,"[3] though in the flux of performance, Lady Saw does vacillate between "out" and "in" and between the definite and the possessive articles.[4] Lake's literal-minded reading of the "sexist" lyrics of the song entirely misses the metaphorical elements that highlight the intense pleasure of vigorous, not violent, sex. The penis here functions as a metaphorical dagger stabbing pleasure into and out of the woman. Conventional associations of orgasm and death in western culture are just as applicable to Jamaican dancehall culture.

Furthermore, the startling imagery of stabbing meat, whether in or out, is decidedly *not* a sign of Lady Saw's sadomasochism but rather underscores the traditional association between food and sex in Caribbean culture. The vivid image is an accurate representation of the way in which meat is seasoned in Caribbean cookery: it is literally pricked and the spices inserted. The metaphor of the woman's genitalia as meat doubles the pleasure of eating, though in this song Lady Saw, like most male DJs declares that she, herself, refuses to eat "fur burger." Despite the recurring protestations in the lyrics of the DJs that they do not "bow"—that is engage in oral sex—one instinctively knows that they are protesting too much. There is a thin line between pub(l)ic discourse and private pleasure/duty.[5]

So what sounds to Obiagele Lake's unseasoned North American ears like abuse of the female body can be reinterpreted from a Caribbean perspective as an X-rated affirmation of the pleasures of heightened sexual passion:

Mi hear you can grind good and can fuck straight.

Stab out mi meat, stab out mi meat.

The big hood [penis] you have a mad gal outa street.

Stab out mi meat.[6]

Lake chastises not only Lady Saw but also those of us fans who pay careful attention to the full range of the DJ's lyrics and know that she is not a one-dimensional artist who uncritically reproduces sexist norms.

In addition to the sexually explicit songs for which she is infamous, Lady Saw's repertoire includes impeccable hymns, country and western laments, songs of warning to women about the wiles of men and politically "conscious" lyrics that constitute hardcore socio-cultural analysis. Failing to understand the complexity of Lady Saw's anansi *persona* and thus her appeal to a wide cross-section of intelligent fans, a bemused Obiagele Lake totally dismisses the recuperative reading of the body of woman in dance-hall culture that is offered by both Inge Blackman and myself in the 1994 Isaac Julien film, *The Darker Side of Black:* ". . . it is perplexing how scholars can honor dance hall music and dance hall behaviors that graphically devalue women since this behavior is nothing more than a continuation of women's objectification. Popular culture critic Carolyn Cooper (1993) condones misogynist lyrics as well as women's lascivious behaviors on the dance floor."[7]

Of course, I do no such thing. I celebrate Lady Saw's entertaining and instructive lyrics, which *Lake* devalues as "misogynist"; and I valorize the erotic dancing that she disdains as "lascivious." I make my own position absolutely clear in the Julien/Gopaul film:

I see the dancehall as a female fertility rite. So that the female body is the central figure in dancehall. If you go to the dance hall you see there's a space where men are very much on the periphery. They're on the margins watching women parade. And people tend to see the female body displayed in very revealing clothes, very short skirts . . . as negative, as the female body is on display as an object. And some people see this transgression, women going outside the bounds of convention that say, you know, that women are the ones who must be responsible for morality and so on. And so this transgressive projection of the body by women I see as something positive – a way of African women asserting the beauty of their bodies in a culture where Black women's bodies are not valued.[8]

In response, Lake launches an amusing line of *ad feminam* attack: "Film director Inge Blackman expresses similar sentiments in Gopaul's film. What is interesting about these views is that it is very unlikely that either Cooper or Blackman would ever appear scantily dressed, performing sexual shows like the women they describe."[9]

The pertinence of Lake's assumptions about my own sartorial preferences and sexual proclivities entirely escapes me. Nevertheless, for the record, let me unashamedly confess that I once performed in a sexual show—even if not as the primary object/subject on display—and thoroughly enjoyed myself. A few years ago I attended a male strip show at Carlos' Café in Kingston. I was invited to experience a lap dance with one Mr. Well Hung, whose day job was barbering in Ocho Rios. He certainly knew how to cut it. Having teased me in my seat, the stripper then pulled me on stage and engaged me in protracted role-play as we danced rub-a-dub style, much to the pleasure of the audience. I certainly know how to distinguish between entertainment, plain and simple, and misogyny. Or, in this case, misandry, to coin a word for the equivalent "hatred" of man—as expressed in the objectification of the male body, put on display for the purely visual pleasure of the female.

Lake concludes her reprimand in this way: "Moreover, Cooper's analysis of the issue of sexism is extremely narrow since it does not address the fact that most people see women *only* in terms of their bodies. Behaving in extremely sexual ways—often to attract men—does nothing to alter this fact."[10] I must question the authority of that all-encompassing generalization that "most people" fail to acknowledge the fact that woman is more than mere meat. Furthermore, in this "screwed-up" reading of gender politics, sexual attraction between men and women is constructed as entirely pathological. Old-fashioned "sex appeal" becomes newfangled neurosis. But, surely, the pleasure that men and women share in sexual relationships of mutual trust can be acknowledged as therapeutic, not exploitative. Self-righteous critics of the sexualized representation of women in Jamaican dancehall culture, who claim to speak unequivocally on behalf of "oppressed" women, often fail to acknowledge the pleasure that women themselves consciously take in the salacious lyrics of both male and female DJs who affirm the sexual power of women.

I do concede that, as Lake rightly observes, commercial sex workers (both male and female) are often disempowered, caught in a cycle of exploitation from which escape is difficult: "Women have been undressing for men in theaters and bars for centuries—the more they take off, the more they shake and gyrate, the more pleasure men receive. This is not new. Indeed, if liberation were as simple as disrobing, exposing yourself in public, and having public sex, women would have been free long ago."[11] But not all consensual adult sex in the dancehall can be reduced to the lowest common commercial denominator. Indeed, in the film *Dancehall Queen,* a pointed contrast is established between Larry's phallocentric sex shop, where working women glide up and down a rigid pole, and the much more fluid space of the dancehall, where "loose" women enjoy the pleasures of uninhibited display.

I propose that Lady Saw's erotic performance in the dancehall can be recontextualized within a decidedly African diasporic discourse as a manifestation of the spirit of female fertility figures such as the Yoruba Oshun. In *Carnival of the Spirit,* African American Yoruba priestess and cultural activist Luisah Teish characterizes Oshun in this way: "She is Maiden, Mother, and Queen. Yoruba folklore attributes many powers to her. She has numerous lovers and is known by many praise-names. . . . She is the personification of the Erotic in Nature. It is she who sits as Queen of the Fertility Feast."[12] In Jamaica, Oshun reappears as the River Mumma of folklore and religion, both myal and revival.[13] She is described by the Reverend Banbury in his 1894 book, *Jamaican Superstitions, or the Obeah Book,* as "the water spirit—the diving duppy."[14] He notes the reverential appreciation of her aquatic fertility: "She is believed to inhabit every fountainhead of an inexhaustible and considerable stream of water in Jamaica. For this reason the sources of such streams were worshipped, and sacrifices offered. . . ."[15]

Nigerian cultural critic Bibi Bakere-Yusuf proposes yet another female orisha, Oya, as a model for the performance of female sexual identity in the African diaspora. In e-mail correspondence she suggests:

> Oya is not only a river goddess as most female orishas are in that part of the world, she is also the orisha of wind, tornado and, for our purpose (that is the exploration into cultural practices) the orisha of masquerades and female power. One of the things that continues to fascinate me about women in dancehall culture is their use of the mask, spectacle and the assertion of female power in all its diversities and complexities. Bearing in mind that in the Yoruba language the word for Spectacle—*Iron*—is the same for ancestor, the masquerade is a spectacle that celebrates the ancestors, the living and the yet to come. Oya is the deity of the *Egun Egun* (ancestral) masquerade, as well as of spectacle. You can imagine what a fuller exploration into this will mean for theorising cultural expressions such as dancehall and other African diasporic cultures. Oya is the orisha that always springs to mind when I think about dancehall woman.[16]

In her elaboration of Yoruba metaphysics, Nigerian sociologist Oyeronke Oyewumi refines the reading of Oya as a female deity, arguing that the Yoruba language "does not make gender assignations of character or personality."[17] She observes that "Ọya, the Yorùbá female river god (not goddess, because the term *òrìṣà* in Yoruba is not gendered). . . . is usually portrayed as fearsome and ruthless; one of the lines from her praise poetry reads, *'Obìnrin gbona, ọkùnrin sa'* (literally: females will hit the road, and males will run; everybody flees when she appears). This hardly supports the Western idea of femininity."[18]

Both Oshun and Oya are here invoked to inform my reading of female agency in Jamaican dancehall culture. Teish elaborates Oshun's contradictory *moral* qualities in the African diaspora, with particular reference to Brazil and Cuba. Her delineation of the Oshun madonna-whore complex seems entirely relevant to my analysis of the contradictory representations of female sexuality in Jamaican dancehall culture, though I do question the characterization of Oshun as "pagan" with its conventionally negative associations of heathenism:

In Brazil and Cuba, African religion merged with Catholicism and the image of the Goddess was greatly affected. In this hemisphere She has been identified with Mary and suffers from the Madonna-Whore complex. She is referred to as La Puta Santa (the Whore Saint) and envisioned as a prostitute of interracial ancestry. Or She may be known as Yeye Kari (Mother of Kindness) and represented by the statue of the Virgin Mary. These appellations speak more to the cultural and political history of these countries than to the power of the Goddess. For She is a virgin but not in the Catholic sense. She is a virgin in the pagan sense—a woman who belongs to Herself and who is free to interact with whomever She chooses. By identifying Her with Mary, "New World" devotees became ashamed of Her promiscuity in folklore and misunderstood the power of Her intercourse. She has, in many places, simply been reduced to a coquette. But in reality She is Iyalode![19]

Furthermore, the respectful salutation "mumi" [mother], which is routinely given by Jamaican men even to women who are clearly their junior, is evidence of the valorization of the female as nurturer—both maternal and erotic. Indeed, the "belly" from which the child comes and to which the man returns frequently to come and come again—this time from the other end—is both a pleasurable and potentially terrifying space that demands the man's loving attention. In the words of Shabba Ranks:

Yu spend nine months inna belly an yu ha fi go back
Every man ha fi love a uman fi a natural fact
Loving up a woman an yu naa dress back [you won't back off]
Mek sure yu can give di uman di flesh axe[20]

In addition, the moral censure invested in, and provoked by, those Jamaican "bad" words that allude to female genitalia and the bloody specifics of menstruation suggests the potency of female sexuality in the culture. The female aperture, the menstrual blood, the protective cloths, the birthing canal that are alluded to in so many Jamaican "bad" words acknowledge the dread that the regenerative power of the woman often engenders. It is this embodied knowledge of female authority that is invoked in the act of voicing the damning "bad" word: *pussy hole, blood claat* [cloth], *raas claat, bombo-claat.* In the words of that iconoclastic genius Peter Tosh:

> . . . when me say "bombo-claat", a guy wan [wants to] tell me say me mouth is dirty and I'm using "indecent language". And under no sector of laws or constitution can a guy show me or clarify to me why is it this word is indecent. A guy say "damn you", "fuck you" and a guy don't say nothing! But as a man say "bombo-claat" him vex. It has too much spirituality. Is the effectiveness that the word has. Me have a song name "O Bombo-Claat" which me sing, and me sing it with dignity. Seen? If you listen to the song, from the first verse to the last, me wrote so many verses to clarify my song, because me know our middle-class nice, decent, clean people out there don't like that. But they do the most devious and evilous bombo-claat things in the society that even the Devil himself is ashamed of, but them don't wan hear me say bombo-claat. A can't tek dat.[21]

Conventional definitions of spirituality, dignity, and decency are clearly undermined in Tosh's revisionist, *bombo-claat* philosophy.

The *Dictionary of Jamaican English* (*DJE*) defines "raas" as "buttocks" and elaborates: "The word is more often used, however, in an

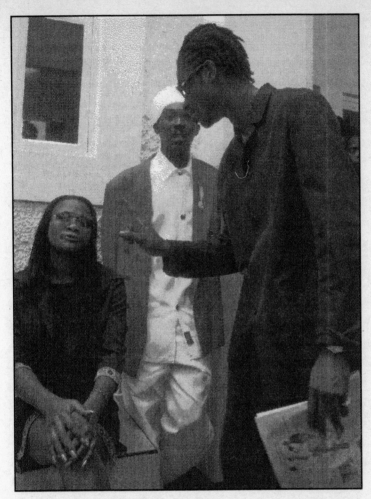

DJs Lady Saw, Anthony B (center), and Bounty Killer, in discussion shortly before they appeared in court to answer to charges of using indecent language during their August 19, 2001 performance at the "Champions in Action" stage show at Fort Clarence Beach, St. Catherine. Photo: Rudolph Brown.

exclamatory way to show strong opposition: scorn, anger, impatience, etc. It is considered very vulgar." The entry on "bumbo" in the *DJE* proposes that the word is "prob[ably] of multiple derivation[s]" and cites Eric

Partridge's 1949 *Dictionary of Slang and Unconventional English:* "Bumbo, occ[asionally] bombo . . . mid-C 18-18, West Indian; orig[inally] a negroes' word." The *DJE* also notes, "African origin is also claimed in the earliest quot[ation] (1774), and cf [compare] Zulu - *bumbu,* pubic region. However, there has prob[ably] been concurrent infl[uence] of English *bum* and perh[aps] also Amer[ican] Sp[anish] *bombo,* both meaning the buttock, rump." The *DJE* also defines bumbo as "[t]he female pudend." The Latin word "pudenda," meaning "that of which one ought to be ashamed," intimates that sexuality is constructed as essentially shameful in eurocentric discourses. Conversely, the brazen use of feminized "bad" words in Jamaican popular culture becomes a subversive reclamation of the contested power of the "bad" and the "vulgar."

In his 1956 study of African-derived Convince religious ceremonies in Jamaica, anthropologist Donald Hogg documents songs performed by "Bongo Men" to summon ancestral spirits. These men, according to Hogg, "believe that spiritual power is morally neutral—that it can be put to both constructive and malevolent purposes by spirits who have it and by persons who can influence them."[22] Some of these Convince songs celebrate "pum-pum"—female genitalia—and its deadly power. Citing a line from one of these songs, "Pum-pum kill me dead, I make he kill me," Hogg offers this interpretation: "[It] concerns the insatiable sexual appetites of Bongo spirits. Freely translated it means, 'If too much sexual intercourse will kill me, then I'll just have to let it kill me.'"[23] Hogg's literal-minded value judgment about "insatiable sexual appetites" seems to miss the point. The song appears to be a metaphorical acknowledgment of the efficacy of pum-pum even for dis/embodied Bongo spirits, which, though already "dead," reclaim materiality through the possession of devotees.

Hogg cites another Convince song in which the spirits beg for pum-pum:

(Chorus)	(Verse)
Whole-a-night (all night)	Me da beg him mother-in-law

Whole-a-night	Me da beg him little more
Whole-a-night	Me da beg him father-in-law
Whole-a-night	Me a want a little more
Whole-a-night	Me da beg him little pum-pum.
Whole-a-night	Me da beg him more and more.[23]

In Jamaican, "him" signifies both male and female. So the verse in English becomes:

I am begging her mother-in-law
I am begging for a little more
I am begging her father-in-law
I want a little more
I am begging her for a little "pum-pum"
I am begging her for more and more

These Convince songs clearly illustrate the potent spirituality of "pum-pum" in African diasporic religion in Jamaica and in its contemporary reconfigurations in dancehall culture.

Trinidadian literary critic and linguist Maureen Warner-Lewis reports her observation of erotic folk dances in Guyana that similarly evoke religious ritual:

During a dance performed in my presence by a women's group in Berbice, Guyana, the leader of the dance circle erotically clapped one hand over her genitals while raising her other hand to clasp the back of her neck, an action also portrayed by some male dancers in the "winding-down" session after the performance of the **beele** "play" in Jamaica. . . . The leader described her action as part of a wedding dance that highlighted the significance of fertility; while making her gesture she exclaimed the word **bombo**, a reference to the female genitals, a word much used in Jamaica as an obscenity, and which has several Central African sources: the Bembe and

Nyanga **mbombo ~ bombo** "anus, arse," the related Koongo near-synonym
bombo "wetness, clotted matter," Mbundu **bombo** "cavity" and, even
more to the point, Mbundu **mbumbu**, "vulva."[25]

Like the dancing female body in Jamaican popular culture, these cognate
Central African words that denote female fertility have undergone pejora-
tion to obscenity in the diaspora.

But Jamaican dancehall DJ philosophers themselves offer alternate
readings of the sexualized female body that reclaim the potency of embodied spirituality. For example, Prezident Brown and Don Yute, declaring the
African genesis of contemporary popular dance in Jamaica, contest the
censorial labeling of erotic dance as "slack." In the song "African Ting"
they assert, combination-style:

Prezident Brown:

It's a African ting so African people sing

And if yu love what yu hear mek me hear yu chanting

Well dem took we foreparents from di mother land

Africa we from an a there we belong

African an Jamaicans we all are one

So mek we beat pon di drum and sing dis ya song

Come een Don Yute come gi yu contribution

Don Yute:

If yu see a gyal a wine [gyrate] pon all her head top

No bother put on no label like di gyal slack

A vibes she a vibes to di sound weh she hear

Is a African ting an she bring it down here

It's a African ting so African people sing

An if you love what yu hear

Mek mi hear yu chanting

All di dance dem weh a cause all a explosion

All a dem a come from inna di motherland

Bogle dancing, butterfly dancing

An di tati dancing

All [even] world-a-dance is a African ting[25]

Prezident Brown's urgent call to "beat pon di drum and sing dis ya song" is a reminder of the outlawing of African languages and musical traditions in the period of slavery. That repressive legacy manifests itself in the Jamaican elite's absolute contempt for the body language of the contemporary dancehall.

In a 1998 radio interview in the "Uncensored" series on Jamaica's Fame FM, Lady Saw audaciously counters charges of vulgarity with coquettish assurance:

Interviewer: Lady Saw, you do things like, yu [you] grab yu crotch on stage. . . .

Lady Saw: Uh huh. Michael Jackson did it and nobody say anything about it.

Interviewer: And you gyrate on the ground. I mean, do you think this is acceptable for a woman?

Lady Saw: Yes, darling. For this woman. And a lot of woman would like to do the same but I guess they are too shy.

Shyness is not one of Lady Saw's obvious attributes/limitations. In response to the question, "Some people are saying that you are vulgar on stage and your lyrics are indecent. Do you think they are justified?" she dismissively asserts: "I think critics are there to do their job and I am here to do my job . . . To entertain and please my fans." And she discounts those critics who naively identify her, Marion Hall, with her stage persona, Lady Saw. She unambiguously declares, "Lady Saw is a act." Pure role-play. Distinguishing between her job and her identity, she claims a private space that allows her the freedom to escape her public image: "I'm a nice girl. When I'm working, you know, just love it or excuse it."

But many critics find it difficult to either love Lady Saw's performances or excuse her transgressions. Most are caught between self-righteous condemnation and open-mouthed fascination. Listen to the ambiguous tone of enthralled reproof in the words of Papa Pilgrim, a reggae radio disc jockey in Salt Lake City, Utah, in his report on the 1993 Reggae Sunsplash "Dancehall Night": "Then came a performance that was more vulgar than any I have seen from anyone anywhere! Her name is Lady Saw, and as a Jamaican friend commented, you cannot put enough Xs in front of her name to adequately describe what she did. To quote from the Aug. 3 *Gleaner,* 'She went to the bottom of the pit and came up with sheer filth and vulgar lyrics which made Yellow Man at his worst seem like a Boy Scout.'"[27]

Exponentially X-rated Lady Saw was not nominated for a Jamaica Music Award for 1994 on the grounds that she is consistently slack. But this is not at all so. The notorious public image of defiant sensuality and raw slackness masks the true depth of Lady Saw's insights, which she reveals, when it suits her, in cutting lyrics that are above reproach. For example, in the sardonic tune "What Is Slackness," Lady Saw interrogates conceptions of slackness that limit the meaning of the word to the private domain of individual sexual transgression. She deconstructs slackness, offering a provocative redefinition that expands the denotative range of the word to include the many failures of the state to fulfill its obligations to the citizenry. In this dancehall subversion, slackness becomes a public matter of communal accountability, and the spotlight of moral judgment is turned away from the DJ herself and on to her detractors:

> Jamaican:
> Want to know what slackness is?
> I'll be the witness to dat.
> Unu come off a mi back.
> Nuff more tings out there want deal with
> An unu naa see dat.
> Society a blame Lady Saw fi di system dem create
> When culture did a clap

Dem never let mi through the gate

As mi say "sex" dem waan fi jump pon mi case

But take the beam outa yu eye

Before yu chat inna mi face

Cause Slackness is

When the road waan fi fix

Slackness when government break them promise

Slackness is when politician issue out gun

And let the two Party a shot them one another down.[28]

English:

Do you want to know what slackness is?

Let me be the witness

You all just get off my back

There are lots of other issues to be dealt with

And you all are not seeing that

Society is blaming Lady Saw

For the system they have created

When culture was all the rage

They wouldn't let me through the gate

I just have to say "sex" and they want to jump on my case

But take the beam out of your eye

Before daring to say anything to me

Because Slackness is roads needing to be fixed

Slackness is the Government breaking its promises

Slackness is politicians issuing guns

And letting Party supporters shoot each other

In a brilliant riposte to her adversaries on her exclusion from the 1994 Jamaica Music Awards competition, Lady Saw recorded a totally unslack hit about the act of censorship. She mockingly asserts that she doesn't need the "award"—the stamp of approval from "certain guys [who] have big position."[29] She is working for the far more valuable "reward" of popularity with her fans. Refusing to be put on pause, she defiantly declares "Mi naa lock mi mout" [I won't lock my mouth]. In deference to the children, though, she carefully edits her lyrics. But you can just imagine the "breed of things" she really wanted to tell the music awards' advisory committee:

Jamaican:

Chorus

Them ha fi bun mi out fi get mi out

No matter wa dem try, mi naa lock mi mout

Dem waan mi fi resign

But it's not yet time

Mi gwy bother dem nerves

And pressure them mind.

Verse 1

If it wasn't for the sake of the children

Some breed a tings mi wuda tell them!

But just because of mi commitment

I'm standing firm to please my audience.

Mi tell dem "Slackness" but it seems dem ears cork

Dem a try and a die fi put mi pon "pause"

Verse 2

A no notn if mi no inna dem roll call

Mek dem keep dem award

Mi a wok fi reward

Through certain guys have big position

Dem fling mi out of dem nomination

But that alone can't stop mi from nyam

The more dem fight, the more mi get strong.

English:

Chorus

They have to burn me out to get me out

No matter what they try, I'm not going to shut up

They want me to resign

But it's not yet time

I'm going to bother their nerves

And keep up the pressure

If it wasn't for the children

I would tell them all kinds of things!

But just because of my commitment

I'm standing firm to please my audience.

I gave them "Slackness" but it seems that their ears are closed

They are trying their hardest to put me on "pause"

Verse 2

It's no big deal if I'm not in their roll call

Let them keep their award

I'm working for my reward

Because certain guys are influential

They have flung me out of their nomination

But that alone can't stop me from earning a living

The more they fight against me, the stronger I get.

The hotter the battle, the sweeter the victory. And sanctified Lady
Saw knows her Bible. You had better take the beam out of your own eye
before you start looking for the mote in hers. In a wicked reversal of roles,
the persecuted DJ sings triumphant praises to God:

When I remember where I'm coming from

Through all the trials and tribulation

Yes, the hardship and the sufferation

I have to go on my knees

And sing praises to God

Glory be to God!

Praises to his name!

Thanks for taking me

Out of the bondage and chains.[30]

Lady Saw proves that she is not consistently slack; she can be as pious as pious can be. And, in any case, she knows that the man from Galilee had a way with all kinds of ladies. So she has quite a few songs in her repertoire that are straight hymns, celebrating divine guidance in her life, and she is quite pragmatic in matters of religion. In that "Uncensored" interview she makes it clear that economic priorities dictate her lifestyle at present. But she doesn't rule out the possibility of conversion to religious respectability at a more convenient season. It is this kind of contradiction that makes Lady Saw such a fascinating character.

In this same spirit of moral ambivalence Lady Saw refuses to set up herself as a role model for young girls who may not have the fortitude and self-possession she displays. And, most often, they are not sophisticated enough to distinguish between role play and reality:

Interviewer: Lady Saw, you said not so long ago that you wouldn't want your daughter to do what you're doing now. What would you say to a young girl now out there who wants to be nothing but just like you?

Lady Saw: I tell them all the time [when] them come to me with it, "I want to be like you Lady Saw." "Like me? You choose sopn [something] else." I can tek [take] my consequences dem right now. I don't know if she strong enough to deal with what I'm dealing with. So I don't encourage them to be like Lady Saw. Sometimes they say, "I love all yu [your] songs." I seh [say], "Yu try listen to the good ones, not the bad ones."

The vast majority of songs in Lady Saw's repertoire are decidedly raunchy. There is no denying it. That is why she is so popular. She is a woman running neck and neck with the men, giving as good, or even better, than she gets. But exclusive focus on those X-rated lyrics diminishes the range of her contribution. Consider, for example, her "Condom" hit, which advocates safe sex. Ironically, Lady Saw is on firm moral ground here. "Condom" is not at all slack—in the usual hard-core sense of the word—though it does name sexual acts/positions that are encoded in metaphor: "banana peel" and "pedal and wheel." The song warns against sexual promiscuity and its fatal consequences. Lady Saw calls attention to the fact that marriage is no guarantee of sexual fidelity, and she recognizes the need to forthrightly negotiate the dangers of sexual intercourse. Playing shy can be a deadly game, and looks can be terminally deceiving:

Jamaican:
Can't know the right and do the wrong
(You see weh me a seh?)
This is reaching out to all woman and man
You see when having sex
Saw beg you use protection (Safety)

Chorus
A condom can save your life (men)
Use it all with your wife (yes)
All when she huff and puff
Tell her without the condom you nah do no wo'k.
Don't bother play shy
Tell the guy, "No bareback ride
No, no, no"
No watch the pretty smile
Remember AIDS will tek you life.[31]

English:

You can't know what's right and do wrong

(You see what I'm saying?)

This is reaching out to all women and men

You see when you're having sex

Saw is begging you to use protection (Safety)

Chorus

A condom can save your life (men)

Use it even with your wife (yes)

And even if she huffs and puffs

Tell her you're not performing without the condom

Don't bother to pretend to be shy

Tell the guy, "No bareback ride

No, no, no"

Don't get taken in by the pretty smile

Remember that AIDS will take your life

Lady Saw confidently asserts that this song can't be banned. Its message is above reproach:

Jamaican:

Them have fe play this one

This one caan get ban

I predict this will be my next number one

Reaching out to teenagers, woman and man

When having sex use protection[32]

English:

They have to play this one

This one can't be banned

I predict that this will be my next number one

Reaching out to teenagers, women and men

Use protection whenever you have sex

Lady Saw comments on changing patterns of sexual behavior that make new precautions imperative. In a clever play on words, the precaution of the condom becomes extended to encompass all the other precautions that must now be taken. In the absence of a commitment to monogamy, sexually active men and women—regardless of social class—are forced to concede the dangers of promiscuity:

Jamaican:

Dem say one man to one woman

That nah gwaan again,

So take precaution

It no matter where you live or who you are

You could be a millionaire or a superstar

We all are one

Come mek we sit down[33]

English:

They say one man for one woman

Is a thing of the past

So take precautions

It doesn't matter where you live or who you are

You could be a millionaire or a superstar

We all are one

Come, let's talk about it.

The DJ's precautionary warnings do not conform to the expectations of what a promiscuous performer like Lady Saw is supposed to advocate. Indeed, a song like "Condom" contests the stereotypes of the dancehall as a hotbed of sensuality from which all reason has fled. Lady Saw challenges her audience to take seriously her warnings about the dangers of casual sex. It is no laughing matter:

> Jamaican:
> When I'm talking don't you dare laugh!
> If them say that Matey a rebel
> So check yourself before you wreck yourself
> No bother move like Mantel and the gal Sketel
> Safety first and trust go to hell[34]

> English:
> Don't you dare laugh when I'm talking!
> If they say the "other woman" is rebelling
> So check yourself before you wreck yourself
> Don't get on like a loose man or woman
> Safety first and trust can go to hell

Acknowledging the feelings of embarrassment that might make some people shy about openly buying condoms, Lady Saw wittily contrasts that instinct for privacy with the public exposure—as on the *Oprah Winfrey* show—that is a potential consequence of not taking precautions:

> Jamaican:
> Instead of saying if you did know
> Go pick you condom at the corner store
> Nobody's business,
> The world nah fi know
> No make sake a hard ears
> You name and face
> Gone pon Oprah talk show.[35]

English:

Instead of having to say "if only I'd known"

Go and select your condoms at the corner store

It's nobody's business

The world doesn't have to know

Don't let stubbornness cause

Your name and face

To be exposed on Oprah's talk show

Lady Saw then goes to the meat of the matter. Naming popular sexual acts/positions, she pointedly asks if sex is worth dying for:

Jamaican:

How do you feel

When you get you banana peel

The wickedest slam

To make you pedal and wheel

Only to find out that you have AIDS disease

You no want know, so get you condom please[36]

English:

How would you feel

When you get your banana peeled

The most exciting sex

That makes you pedal and wheel

Only to find out that you have the disease, AIDS

You don't want to know, so please get your condoms

Discrediting derogatory references to her supposedly mindless promiscuity, Lady Saw makes a public declaration of her own refusal to engage in sex without taking precautions. She sets up herself as a role model of responsible sexual behavior. And her sense of accountability extends beyond safe sex to the advocacy of a much more generalized program of proper healthcare:

Jamaican:

Some critics say that I am a sex machine

Me no know bout that

This I will reveal

If my man don't put on him rubbers

Him nah be able fi tell the Saw thanks.

When it come to me health, I'm serious

Take me pap smear, mi usual check-up

Then everything fall back in line

If him nah wear no condom

Him nah get no bligh.[37]

English:

Some critics say that I'm a sex machine

I don't know about that

But this is what I can tell you

If my man doesn't put on his condom

He won't have the chance to tell the Saw thanks

When it comes to my health, I'm serious

I do my pap smear and get my regular check-ups

Then everything falls back into place

If he won't wear a condom

He's not getting any.

Lady Saw warns vulnerable young women about the cunning strategies some irresponsible men employ to avoid the use of condoms. She advocates vigilance, not just in the moment of the sex act, but more generally as a strategy for exercising control over one's fate.

Jamaican:

No make dem fool you

That when them use it

Them no feel you

That nuh true, girls.

Some wi want bus' it

When dem put it on

So open yu ears and

Watch what a gwaan.

English:

Don't let them fool you into believing

That when they use it

They don't feel you

That's not true, girls.

Some will try to burst it

When they're putting it on

So open your eyes and

Watch out for what's going on.

Lady Saw's brilliant lyrics, reinforced by her compelling body language, articulate a potent message about sexuality, gender politics, and the power struggle for the right to public space in Jamaica. She is a woman who knows the power of her own sex appeal. As an entertainer, she fully understands the function of performance as a strategy for masking the self. Indeed, erotic disguise extends beyond the dress codes and role-play of the celebrants in the dancehall, as elaborated in the following chapter. It encompasses the cunning strategies that are employed by outspoken women like Lady Saw who speak subtle truths about their society. In the spirit of Oshun, River Mumma, and Oya, Goddess of the Masquerade, Lady Saw cuts loose from the boundaries that would contain her. She is a river of sensuality running free.

FOUR

"Mama, Is That You?"

Erotic Disguise in the Films
Dancehall Queen and *Babymother*

In *Dancehall Queen* and *Babymother*, the film medium becomes a site of transformation in which the spectacularly dressed bodies of women in the dancehall assume extraordinary proportions once projected onto the screen. In both films, one set in Jamaica, the other in the United Kingdom, the styling of the body—the hair, makeup, clothes, and body language that are assumed—enhances the illusion of a fairy-tale metamorphosis of the mundane self into eroticized sex object. The fantastic un/dress code of the dancehall, in the original Greek sense of the word "fantastic," meaning "to make visible," "to show," is the visualization of a distinctive cultural style that allows women the liberty to demonstrate the seductive appeal of the imaginary—and their own bodies. In an elaborate public striptease, transparent bedroom garments become theatrical street wear, somewhat like the emperor's new clothes. And who dares say that the body is naked? Only the naive.

This dancehall affirmation of the pleasures of the body, which is often misunderstood as a devaluation of female sexuality, also can be theorized as an act of self-conscious female assertion of control over the representa-

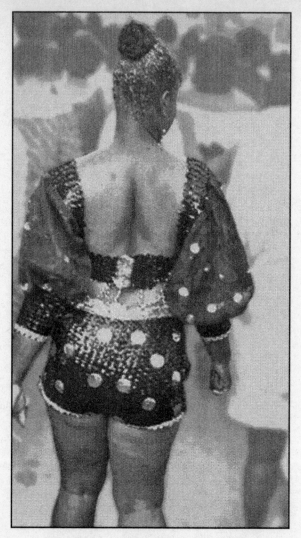

Dancehall funeral dress, 1992. Photo: Winston Sill.

tion of her person. Woman as sexual being claims the right to sexual pleasure as an essential sign of her identity. Both fleshy women and their more sinewy sisters are equally entitled to display themselves in the public sphere as queens of revelry. Exhibitionism conceals ordinary imperfections. In the dancehall world of make-believe, old roles can be contested and new identities assumed. Indeed, the elaborate styling of both hair and clothes is a permissive expression of the pleasures of disguise. In the words of dancehall Diva Sandra Lee: "The extension add a movie look to us. . . . Is like a disguise. I want to look different tomorrow."[1]

The blurb for *Dancehall Queen* locates the film's fairy-tale antecedents in this way: "*Dancehall Queen* is a modern-day Cinderella story, with no Prince Charming, but one very strong woman. . . ."[2] The Caribbean stereotypes of the superhuman Black woman and the delinquent Black man meet the European fantasy of the nurturing Prince Charming; and part company. At the center of *Dancehall Queen* is a disguise drama in which the star, Marcia, outsmarts the Don, Larry, contriving to make him believe that she is other than her everyday self—an unglamorous street vendor, pushing a heavy cart through the streets of Kingston in the unending struggle to survive. She is the work-weary mother of two children, the older of whom, Tanya, is a nubile teenager targeted for sexual abuse by Larry, the predator, disguised as benefactor.

But Marcia is not inspired to assume the dazzling disguise of Dancehall Queen in order to seduce Larry and divert him from her daughter. Nor is it the promise of sex/romance that tempts her, though she does come to enjoy her newly discovered power to arrest Larry's attention that had been so single-mindedly focused on Tanya. It is the prize money, which guarantees a measure of economic independence, however temporary, that motivates Marcia. Furthermore, she is inspired to succeed in her bid for the crown of Dancehall Queen by her recognition of the power of costume to enable the transformation. When Marcia encounters the reigning Dancehall Queen, Olivene, in street clothes and in the glare of daylight, she is struck by the pedestrian quality of the woman. I use "pedestrian" deliberately because in Jamaica, as elsewhere, cars are often marketed as a fashion accessory that can add immeasurable style to their owner/occupant, somewhat like Cinderella's pumpkin chariot.[3]

The glittering strobe-light world of the dance is an idealized space in which fantastic identities are possible. Once out of costume, the glamorous fairy-tale princess/ hard-core Dancehall Queen often loses her appeal. Stripped of accessories, she is put to the test and found wanting. Indeed, Marcia's incredulous and malicious comment about Olivene—"She look[s] ordinary eeh!"—signals her own recognition of the distance between the nocturnal image and the daylight reality. When Marcia herself eventually does win the crown of Dancehall Queen, it is essential that she resume her costume as street vendor to reclaim her own sense of identity. But she thoroughly enjoys the fairy-tale fantasy of hypersexuality that the stage properties of the dancehall engender. Indeed, the persona of "dancehall queen" permits Marcia to savor the sensuality that had been repressed in the drudgery of her everyday existence. As she flaunts the wigs and other accessories so essential to her new role, she is able to attract suitors like the videographer, for whom she becomes the seductive "Mystery Lady."

The camera's eye redefines Marcia as a worthy subject of attention, bedecked in all her borrowed glory. She unashamedly revels in the male gaze. No feminist anxieties of "objectification" disturb her. Indeed, quite early in the game, when the videographer turns his camera away from her to acknowledge the presence of reigning Dancehall Queen Olivine, Marcia gets into a huff. She wants to be the singular focus of the videographer's attention. In an illuminating essay, Maggie Humm observes:

The gaze is both a metaphor in film criticism and an integral part of film discourse and narrative. Laura Mulvey first introduced the idea that men looking at women in film use two forms of mastery over her: a sadistic voyeurism which controls women's sexuality through dominating male characters, and a symbolic fetishisation of women's sexuality. Mulvey shows that cinema enables this male gaze to create the illusion, through a complicated system of point-of-view, that the male spectator is producing the gaze. The male character carries the gaze of the male spectator as his assistant. Women are objectified erotic objects existing in film simply as recipients of the male gaze. The aim, then, for Mulvey is to explain the function of film in the erotic violation of women by revealing its system of voyeuristic pleasure. To Mulvey, feminist directors have only to generate new notions of female sexuality by using *avant-garde* practices of spectator-film relationships in order to deconstruct the scopic gaze.[4]

Humm, conceding in a footnote that Mulvey has "modified her position to give a much more sophisticated account of the gaze," does acknowledge the centrality of the latter's early work in theorizing the gaze. Nevertheless, Humm argues for an even more subtle reading of the politics of spectatorship that recognizes the pleasure that women as agents do take in desiring and being desired:

> Mulvey's criticism has done a lot to help us examine the question of the gendered spectator, yet, because her method derives from psychoanalytic accounts, via Lacan, of the formation of female subjectivity, it allows little scope for analysing female subjectivity in its semiotic or social discourses. Mulvey sets up too rigid a divide between visual analysis and contextual discourse. In any case, psychoanalysis has not dealt adequately with desire, since it does not read sexuality as that which must be continually produced.[5]

In Marcia's case, desire—both hers and that of the videographer—rehumanizes her, putting her at center stage. And even after she is stripped of her disguise, she remains attractive to her videographer. The persona of dancehall queen thus generates residual benefits for Marcia, who now transfers to her "real" life the embodied power that her fantasy had bestowed.

Shape-shifting and mistaken identity are familiar motifs in folktales of many cultures. In the Caribbean, popular stories of both West African and European origin encode disguise dramas. Alice Werner's scholarly introduction to Walter Jekyll's 1907 collection, *Jamaican Song and Story,* concludes with an analysis of five stories classified as of the "Robber

Bridegroom" type, "the Robber being the equivalent of an earlier wizard or devil, who, in the primitive form of the story, was simply an animal assuming human shape." Werner elaborates:

> The main incidents of the type-story are as follows:
>
> (1) A girl obstinately refuses all suitors.
>
> (2) She is wooed by an animal in human form, and at once accepts him.
>
> (3) She is warned (usually by a brother) and disregards the warning.
>
> (4) She is about to be killed and eaten, but is saved by the brother whose advice was disregarded.[6]

Although Werner observes that "[i]n the Jamaican stories it strikes one that the idea of transformation is somewhat obscured," she nevertheless does concede that various disguises *are* assumed by the Robber Bridegrooms to facilitate their duping of the gullible brides. Indeed, Werner notes that "Rabbit," an unsuccessful suitor, "takes no steps to change his shape, being rejected on the ground that he is 'only but a meat,' *i.e.*, an animal."[7]

Dress thus becomes an essential sign of the assumed human identity. Werner summarizes her argument:

> We are told how "Gaulin" (Egret) and "John Crow" provide themselves with clothes and equipages—the latter a carriage and pair, the former the humbler buggy:—and this seems to constitute the extent of the disguise. Yellow Snake is said to "change and fix up himself"—but the expression is vague. Gaulin, however, can only be deprived of his clothes (and so made to appear in his true shape) by means of a magic song. The "old-witch" brother, who has overheard the song, plays its tune at the wedding and thus exposes the bridegroom, who flies out the door. "John-Crow" is detected by a Cinderella-like device of keeping him til daylight, and his hurried flight through the window (in which he scraped the feathers off his head on the broken glass) explains a characteristic feature of these useful but unattractive birds.[8]

Contemporary dancehall culture in Jamaica discloses new variants of the shape-shifting motifs that are inscribed in traditional folktales. Assuming the disguises of dancehall aesthetics, empresses of style like Marcia can fulfill complicated sexual fantasies. Like the animals of folktale that deploy human dress to seduce the objects of their desire, marginalized working-class Black women in Jamaica now assume the habits of seduction to full advantage. For example, in the putting on of wigs, weaves, and extensions in various hues, "picky-picky head" women go to all lengths to claim the sex appeal that is perceived to reside naturally in "tall-hair" women, as evidenced in the dominant images of pinup female sexiness in the mainstream media in Jamaica and elsewhere.[9]

Hairpieces do for some women what dreadlocks and the even more fashionable "sisterlocks" do for others. Although length and volume of store-bought hair are valorized, height is also crucial and adds another layer of constructed beauty that bears absolutely no resemblance to contemporary eurocentric modes of hairstyling. Dancehall hairstyles are engineered and require sophisticated technical skills for their construction. Indeed, this dancehall hair-extension aesthetic must be acknowledged as a contemporary expression of traditional patterns of hair and body adornment in continental Africa, which have now gloriously reemerged in the diaspora. As they flash their Rapunzel tresses, these dancehall divas appropriating the border-crossing potential of disguise simultaneously reinscribe and subvert the racial ideology that devalues the "natural" beauty of African Jamaican women and undermines their self-esteem.

In an entertaining and instructive ethnographic study, Ingrid Banks confronts the subject of the politics of hair head-on. In the chapter "Splitting Hairs: Power, Choice and Femininity," she documents the voices of women who assert their right to self-definition and identifies the often-contradictory politics of liberation that is manifested in the hairstyling choices of African American women and, by extension, their Caribbean sisters:

An important critique of the self-hatred account of hair alteration is that it does not take into consideration hairstyling practices that reflect how black women exercise power and choice, as some women noted in chapter 2 ["The Hair 'Do's' and 'Don'ts' of Black Womanhood"]. The possibility that hairstyling practices, in whatever form, serve as a challenge to mainstream notions of beauty or that they allow black women to embrace a positive identity is important for two reasons: voice and empowerment. Voice is important for marginalized groups in U.S. society, and it is through voice that black women are not merely victims of oppression. Instead, black women are agents or thinking and acting beings who understand the forces that shape their lives.[10]

In the words of Flip Wilson, that irreverent African American wit, "When you look good, you feel good; and when you feel good, you move good."

A similarly sophisticated reading of the makeup practices of Black women must take into account the many shades of meaning that the brush paints. In some instances, makeup does function explicitly to mask/erase distinctly "African" features. Techniques for reducing the width of the nose, for example, require a subtle play of light and shade to highlight the bridge of the nose and downplay the surrounding flesh. Nevertheless, there is an element of pure artistry and empowering aesthetic pleasure in the practice of making up that should not be denigrated. Writing out of the inter/discipline of British fashion studies, Catherine Constable, like Ingrid Banks, underscores conceptions of the mask of makeup "as that which foregrounds its own constructedness and therefore possesses a kind of truthfulness."[11] In the conclusion to her fascinating essay "Making Up the Truth: On Lies, Lipstick and Friedrich Nietzsche," she elaborates this argument:

Once the mask is not viewed as purely patriarchal, or merely indicative of the absence of truth, it becomes a construct that can be mobilised in a variety of ways. This means that the mask can be seen to generate a wide variety of possible meanings rather than simply and reductively indicating its status as "untruth" or the "untruth of truth." Furthermore, the analysis of the mask as truthful clearly has important implications for feminism in that it radically destabilises the definition of glamour as objectification. This creates a space for thinking about the radical potential of the power to hold the gaze and the ways in which that power might be instantiated by a range of female icons.[12]

The title of Banks's book clearly signifies on Cornel West's *Race Matters*. It thus asserts that what is essentially a feminized discourse—the politics of Black hair—demands just as much critical attention as those more conventional domains in which the racialized politics of identity is addressed—such as in the predominantly masculine arena of sports. By thus equating "race" and "hair," Banks elevates a "woman's" issue to the center of discourse. If race matters, hair matters as much because hair marks socially constructed racial difference. In the "Introduction: Unhappy to be Nappy," Banks observes, "The research presented in the following pages is not about hair per se. *Hair Matters* illustrates how hair shapes black women's ideas about race, gender, class, sexuality, images of beauty, and power."[13]

Cornel West's argument about the perverse consequences of racist representations of the Black body in the American imaginary is especially acute when applied to Black women. Though West's choice of "refusal" unconscionably intimates that the victim willfully embraces denigration, he nevertheless accurately delineates the history of trauma:

... [M]uch of black self-hatred has to do with the refusal of many black Americans to love their black bodies—especially their black noses, hips, lips, and hair. Just as many white Americans view black sexuality with disgust, so do many black Americans—but for different reasons and with different results. White supremacist ideology is based first and foremost on the degradation of black bodies in order to control them. One of the best ways to instill fear in people is to terrorize them. Yet this fear is best sustained by convincing them that their bodies are ugly, their intellect is inherently underdeveloped, their culture is less civilized, and their future warrants less concern than that of other peoples.[14]

In the patriarchal politics of most societies, women are required to be beautiful, unlike men, who are allowed to be their natural selves, however ugly. In the derisory words of the self-important male character Ubana in the novel *The Joys of Motherhood,* written by the Nigerian Buchi Emecheta: "A woman may be ugly and grow old, but a man is never ugly and never old. He matures with age and is dignified."[15] For many African diasporan women, the politics of beauty is complicated by racism. Unlike their African sisters, for whom beauty was traditionally defined in indigenous terms, many African women in the diaspora are judged by standards of beauty based on non-African phenotypes. Faced with these marks of erasure, many African diasporan women have had to settle for being sexy instead of beautiful.

There is an old Guyanese joke about an African Guyanese entrant in a beauty contest in the mid-1960s. The story was told to an African Guyanese woman who worked at Fogarty's, a Georgetown store that tended to have a disproportionately high percentage of Portuguese and other light-skinned employees. The unsuccessful beauty contestant is alleged to have responded thus to a malicious question about how she fared in the competition:

> For figure and face
> I ain't mek no place
> But for bubby an arse
> Ah bus deh rass.[16]

Not all African diasporan women share the confidence of this contestant. In fact, the beauty contest culture in Jamaica, for example, still privileges the "browning" and occasionally the "white" woman as the ideal phenotype to represent this "out of many, one people" nation in international beauty competitions.

Furthermore, there is a disturbing trend in the Caribbean today for Black women to bleach their skin in an attempt to approximate the standards of Euro-American ideal beauty, especially its mulatto variant. This bleaching of the skin—usually only the face and neck—is an obvious attempt to partially disguise the racial identity of the subject. The mask of "lightness," however dangerous in medical terms, becomes a therapeutic signifier of status in a racist society that still privileges melanin deficiency as a sign of beauty. And there is decided ambivalence about the use of these bleaching agents. Some obvious bleachers, when confronted with the question, "Why yu a bleach?" [Why are you bleaching?], cunningly attempt to conceal the evidence. A recurring explanation for the "coolness" of the skin is the claim "is because mi work in aircondition office." This adds yet another layer of disguise to the subject, for many such respondents may, in fact, be unemployed.

For me, the most alluring account of this refusal to admit that one is bleaching the skin comes from a young woman who sells in Kingston's Papine Market, whose face, all of a sudden, began to assume an unusual ghostly whiteness, a vivid contrast with the rest of her body. When I nosily commented on what had happened to her face and asked why she was bothering to bleach, she rather airily informed me that I was mistaking her for her sister. Now, it is true that this young woman does have a sister who is a little darker than she, and who sometimes sells in the market too. But I know them both well enough not to confuse them. An equally nosy man who works in the market observed in a stage whisper, "Is because she know seh she spoil up herself mek she a tell yu bout a her 'sister'" [It's because she knows that she's spoiled herself why she's telling you that she's her "sister"]. In this young woman's case, role-play manifested a clear desire to deny her basic identity. She has since stopped bleaching, her natural skin color has returned and every now and then I jokingly ask her how her sister is doing. She laughs—with me, I hope.

It is not only women who feel obliged to wear the mask, as the following anecdote illustrates. A panel discussion was held in December 1999 at the Mona Common Basic School where students in the Caribbean Institute of Media and Communication at the University of West Indies were screening a video on bleaching that they had made as part of a research project on the theme "Love the Skin You're In." At the event, a young man who had participated in the study acknowledged the fact that bleaching was harmful to the skin and said he was planning to stop. But he is a DJ who knows the value of looking good on his own terms. Let me recount his explanation, not quite verbatim, but as best as I can recall it, for why he would continue to bleach for a little while longer: "Christmas a come an mi ha fi look good. Mi a go gwaan bleach. An when yu see mi ready fi go out, mi a go put on one long sleeve ganzie and wear mi cap. An dem wi tink a one browning a come through" [Christmas is coming and I have to look good. I'm going to continue bleaching. And when I'm ready to go out, I'm going to put on a long-sleeved jersey and wear my cap. And they will think that it's a browning coming through].

First of all, I felt perversely obliged to disabuse the young man of that fantasy. No one, I told him, would ever mistake him for a browning. And, in any case, he needed to look in the mirror and see that he was perfectly handsome as a Black person. Shades of Michael Jackson hover gloomily in the colonized imagination. In *Flyboy in the Buttermilk,* cultural critic Greg Tate gives a "fanciful" and "empathetic" rereading of the psychology of skin bleaching in a chapter entitled "I'm White!: What's Wrong with Michael Jackson":

> There are other ways to read Michael Jackson's blanched skin and disfig-
> ured African features than as signs of black self-hatred become self-mutila-
> tion. Waxing fanciful, we can imagine the boy-who-would-be-white a
> William Gibson-ish work of science fiction: harbinger of a trans-racial
> tomorrow where genetic deconstruction has become the norm and Narcis-
> sism wears the face of all human Desire. Musing empathetic, we may put the

question, who does Mikey want to be today? The Pied Piper, Peter Pan, Christopher Reeve, Skeletor, or Miss Diana Ross? Our Howard Hughes? Digging into our black nationalist bag, Jackson emerges a casualty of America's ongoing race war—another Negro gone mad because his face does not conform to the Nordic ideal.

To fully appreciate the sickness of Jackson's savaging of his African physiognomy you have to recall that back when he wore the face he was born with, black folk thought he was the prettiest thing since sliced sushi.[17]

Though I am amused by Tate's conflicted reading of Michael Jackson—"Jackson and I are the same age, damn near 30, and I've always had a love-hate thing going with the brother[18]—in retrospect, I do seriously wonder about the appropriateness of my intended reprimand to my skin-bleaching DJ. Not just the issue of my bad manners in pointing out the obvious, but more so the haunting question of whether the young man's understanding of what he was doing was much more sophisticated than I was willing to allow at that time. What remains so fascinating in his narrative is his rather practical sense of seasonal brownness. He knew that being brown, however achieved, was not really an essential part of his identity. Light skin color was a fashion accessory that would stand him in good stead during the festive season. Somewhat like the bright lights that decorate the Christmas landscape, light skin color, however fleeting, would give the DJ added visibility. The metaphor thus underscores both the elements of fantasy as well as the conscious awareness of role-play that are so subtly intertwined in these dancehall discourses of desire.

Furthermore, the DJ's metaphor of "coming through" signals his conception of the color line as a barrier that must be literally breached, so that he can become socially visible. And it takes a lot of cunning, Anansi style, to make the breakthrough possible. Rupturing categories, role-play thus both emancipates and imprisons the "real" self. In the words of Nigerian cultural critic Bibi Bakere-Yusuf, "The black skin (or the 'racial epidermal schema' as [Frantz] Fanon calls it) becomes the sign of radical otherness, of impurities and degeneracy, within the European imaginary. However, through numerous efforts, the skin has often become the very vehicle by which epidermal negation is confronted, contested and negotiated by black people, in order to (re)assert their own humanity."[19]

This predilection for playing the other—that is, "playing mas"—underscores a hidden continuity between the annual rituals of carnival masquerading in other Caribbean societies and the daily gestures of dissimulation in real-time Jamaican culture and its heightened forms of expression in the dancehall. The importation of an adulterated Trinidad carnival aesthetic into Jamaican popular culture has resulted in the cross-fertilization of traditions of role-play in which costume, dance, and music are primal signifiers. And just as the Byron Lee carnival aesthetic creates a platform for predominantly upper/middle-class brown and white Jamaicans to seemingly abandon respectability, parade their nakedness in the streets, and "get on bad" (i.e., pass for Black), on their terms, even so everyday Jamaican dancehall culture permits the Black majority to enjoy the pleasures of release from the prison of identity that limits the definition of the person to one's social class and color.

There are, it is all too true, profound psychosociological underpinnings of this desire to be/play the other that cannot be simply written off as mere entertainment. Role-play both conceals and reveals deep-seated anxieties about the body that has been incised with the scarifications of history. Half a century later, Frantz Fanon's 1952 *Black Skin, White Masks* remains the classic account of this dehumanizing process and its subversion:

> For several years certain laboratories have been trying to produce a serum for "denegrification"; with all the earnestness in the world, laboratories have sterilized their test tubes, checked their scales, and embarked on researches that might make it possible for the miserable Negro to whiten himself and thus to throw off the burden of that corporeal malediction. Below the corporeal schema I had sketched a historico-racial schema. The elements

that I used had been provided for me . . . by the other, the white man, who had woven me out of a thousand details, anecdotes, stories.[20]

Echoing Fanon, Bibi Bakere-Yusuf gives an incisive postmodernist reading of the mask of bleaching in African/diasporic cultures:

The erstwhile superior logic of white flesh is critiqued and exposed as part of a wider field of representation and scopic economy that tries to evade and mask its own investment in representation. Skin bleaching is therefore less a blind or bland imitation of an original and more of a practice whereby the original is presented as a construction that can be taken up, reordered, skewed and jammed in a way that becomes meaningful to the agent. For example, the very women who favour bleaching are also concerned to have full and voluptuous bodies—the antithesis of the kind of bodily figure that goes with such a phenotype. In this respect, bleaching skin can be seen as a superficial form of styling, nothing more than an appropriative aestheticisation of a bodily form, a simple borrowing from another representational regime. In this sense, bleaching certainly has little to do with a desire for dancehall women to become that which they are miming. As a superficial form of styling, bleaching can be thought of as another form of adornment, along the same lines as wearing green or pink wigs or wearing latex batty riders.[21]

This "denaturing" impulse in Jamaican dancehall aesthetics is evident not only in the rituals of skin bleaching but also in another alarming new development—the ingestion by some women of the "fowl pill," the hormones used in the highly mechanized production of poultry to accelerate the fattening of the goods for the market. The metaphorical colloquialism "chick," used as a term of endearment for females, becomes all too literal in this context. Short-circuiting the process of getting the "benefits" of eating the hormone-packed chicken itself, some Jamaican women experiment on themselves to construct the *mampi*-size body that is so highly valorized in the culture: large breasts, thighs and bottoms.[22] The dancehall thus constitutes a paradoxical social space in which the "natural" as a marker of identity is both contested and re-instituted and sexuality, especially that of the large-bodied woman, is celebrated with abandon.

Buju Banton celebrates this culturally validated *mampi*-sized body in "Gal You Body Good."[23] Addressing the generic *good body gal*, the DJ enthusiastically declares that fatness is in style. Perennially. Acknowledging the fact that for most Jamaican men it is the full-bodied woman that is the ideal sexual partner—not the somewhat anorexic beauty queen contestant—Buju urges supposedly "underweight" women to take lessons from their betters. But the DJ encourages "maaga" women to increase their body size not just in order to satisfy male desire but also to amass the muscle power that will enable them to vigorously defend themselves against predatory males.[24] It is this nuanced representation of power relations in dancehall culture that is so intriguing: woman as the seeming victim of the male gaze; versus woman as empowered agent. The dancehall thus constitutes a paradoxical social space in which the "natural" as a marker of identity is both contested and reinstituted and sexuality, especially that of the large-bodied woman, is celebrated with abandon.

In *Dancehall Queen,* Marcia's daughter, Tanya, is incredulous when she discovers her mother rehearsing the role of dancehall queen: "Mama, is that you?" The eroticization of motherhood is the ultimate manifestation of the abandonment of traditional definitions of woman as desexualized caregiver. In both *Dancehall Queen* and *Babymother,* motherhood is a condition that conceals the erotic potential of the woman. The sexuality of the older woman that is usually disguised by her role as mother is released in the taking on of the persona of dancehall queen. This re-eroticization of motherhood challenges the presumption that after a certain age and especially after child bearing the woman naturally loses her sex appeal and must be replaced by a younger woman—often her very own daughter in circumstances in which the woman's putative mate is sexually attracted to his supposed stepdaughter.

Somewhat surprisingly in *Dancehall Queen,* the woman is complicit in the sexual exploitation of her daughter. She functions as a pimp, procuring her daughter for Larry. Yet another layer of disguise: It is her concern for her family's economic well-being that precipitates the decision to sacrifice the daughter. But Tanya is devastated by Larry's predatory desire for her since she views him as a father figure. The enforced sexual relationship that Marcia engineers for her daughter is thus not only rapacious but incestuous. Yet beneath the apparent heartlessness of the mother's action lies a somewhat pragmatic assessment of her daughter's options: Since there is a juvenile suitor in the offing and Tanya seems likely to become sexually active, Marcia figures that her daughter might as well get maximum economic returns on the sexual transaction. Ironically, when Marcia herself convincingly assumes the role of Dancehall Queen, Larry's attention is deflected from Tanya, who is now free to enjoy the innocent pleasures of friendship with her age mate.

In *Babymother,* Anita struggles to claim an identity other than mother. For her the dancehall is a creative space in which another identity as artist can be consummated. As DJ, not mere spectator, she envisions a potential identity that is obscured by the conservative gender ideology that imprisons woman in the role of supportive partner to the male star. Asserting her own power to create lyrics about her reality as babymother, Anita celebrates both her acceptance of the responsibilities of mothering as well as her escape from the constraints that motherhood often imposes on women. As songwriter and performer she is free to reflect on her own experience, thus transforming the burden of mothering into the raw material of art. The glamorization of the male performer is now matched by the glamorization of the babymother as artist.

Anita's babyfather, Don Byron, a reggae superstar, refuses to support her bid to become a star in her own right. He is the quintessential robber bridegroom, the animal in human form, who intends to imprison his babymother in her rightful place within the domestic sphere. He promises

Anita that he will perform a duet with her at a major show and then lets her down, revealing his true colors:

> Byron: A wa yu a do? [What are you doing?] Dis is di place fi di mother of my children. Not di stage. We don't need more than one musician in dis family.
>
> Anita: Hold on! Who are you to tell me how to be a mother? Since when please? Why shouldn't I be out there chatting the mike?
>
> Byron: Cause you're my babymother, that's why.
>
> Anita: What kind of reason is that for anything, yu dyam [damned] fool you?[25]

The pathos of Anita's struggle is intensified by the knowledge that she is valiantly attempting to do what her own mother, Rose, could not: take on the responsibilities of bringing up a child on her own. As in *Dancehall Queen,* in *Babymother* there is an inset disguise drama. For Rose, now a successful solicitor, teenage sexual indiscretion and its usual outcome, pregnancy, had to be disguised in the fiction of indirect affiliation. Not having been offered the expected option of marriage to her delinquent partner, and refusing abortion, the teenage mother chooses the illusion of respectability, a choice that her daughter cannot respect. Rose, passing as her daughter's sister, gives up the child to the care of her own mother because she could not cope with the very conditions of poverty that now circumscribe Anita's life:

> Rose: It was impossible you know. I was so young. Where would we be now? Mom could give you things. You would have just grown up living from hand to mouth. . . .
>
> Anita: On an estate [in the projects] like this? Like Saffron and Anton?
>
> Rose: Listen, Anita, I'm really having a hard time with this.
>
> Anita: And you, a babymother like me. Yeah. Scraping food. Going nowhere.

Rose: No. Yes, but . . .

Anita: I'm busy, Rose.

(Slams door)

Rose's story is an archetypal Caribbean tale. Another popular variant is the mother's disguising herself as her daughter's aunt. For example, in Olive Senior's short story, "Lily, Lily," the truth of the relationship between mother and daughter, both named Lily, is graphically foreshadowed in the daughter's intuitive reconfiguration of the family pictures she scrutinizes, looking for clues to unlock the puzzle. The pun on "gilt" encodes the politics of betrayal that is central to the disguise drama:

> When the thoughts come crowding in she returns to the mama-lily game which she played endlessly as a small child in Mama's room with the high bureau with the pictures she had to climb on a chair to look at. The pictures in the double gilt frame of Mama and Auntie Lily. Mama and Auntie Lily so alike it was hard to tell them apart, so alike when she played the game of looking from one to the other ever so fast her head spun and they merged into the one she saw in the mirror every morning of Lily-the-child, as if she were their child. She felt guilty whenever she thought this, as if she were betraying Mama whom she loved more than anyone in the world. So why, as she got older did she fancy that she looked more like Auntie Lily, wanted more and more to be with Auntie Lillie, become Auntie Lilly?[26]

Despite the stigma attached to teenage pregnancy or, more generally, pregnancy out of wedlock, folk wisdom acknowledges the fact that the very mother who laments the fall of her daughter into premature motherhood, especially if this pregnancy repeats the narrative of her own sexual history, is often seduced into joyous acceptance of the catastrophe when she sees the beautiful child that results. Further, many such women quickly resign themselves to the status of premature grandmotherhood, reclaiming that estate from its conventional associations with decrepitude and asexuality.

In addition, the high level of teenage pregnancy and childbirth among working-class girls in Jamaica and the diaspora is probably matched by the high level of teenage pregnancy and abortion among middle-class girls. Class privilege, which allows varying access to abortion as a moral and economic option, masks the similarity between the sexual practices of working-class and middle-class girls. Many sexually active middle-class girls are protected from the consequences of their actions in ways that are not usually available to working-class girls.

In both *Dancehall Queen* and *Babymother,* erotic disguise functions on various levels. The trope of the "robber bridegroom" is central to my reading of both texts. These films are adapted reinscriptions of traditional folktale in which both bride and groom are now robbers. Both men and women employ subterfuge to best each other. The disguise motif is not limited to the eroticized adornment of the body. Disguise enables the exploration of more profound issues of betrayal as predatory animal nature, unsuccessfully concealed by the mask of the human face, stalks its victims. In both films the female stars are rescued from their robber bridegrooms. But the message of these cautionary tales is not just the fiction of the happy ending. Equally important is the warning that the patterns of seduction and entrapment encoded in folktale are archetypes, surviving in the contemporary dancehall in new guises.

"Lyrical Gun"

Metaphor and Role-Play
in Dancehall Culture

Constant references to guns in Jamaican dancehall lyrics have resulted in an increasing tendency to criminalize the idiom and demonize the culture both locally and in the international marketplace. For example, in a sensational 2002 newspaper article, with the inflammatory headline, "How Dancehall Promotes Violence," Ian Boyne asserts, "There is no way this country can successfully change the culture of violence in the inner cities without changing the culture of the dancehall. We underestimate to our peril the threat of Jamaican dancehall culture to peace."[1] In the equally incendiary follow-up article, "How Dancehall Holds Us Back," Boyne quietly concedes, "It is hard to empirically establish a causal link between murders committed in the inner cities and negative dancehall lyrics."[2] Nevertheless, he finds it quite easy to make the following leap of faith: "But it is not hard to show that these lyrics do not help those people who need to learn how to manage their conflicts and bring about reconciliation."[3] Without offering a shred of evidence, Boyne smugly asserts the validity of his speculations, to his singular satisfaction.

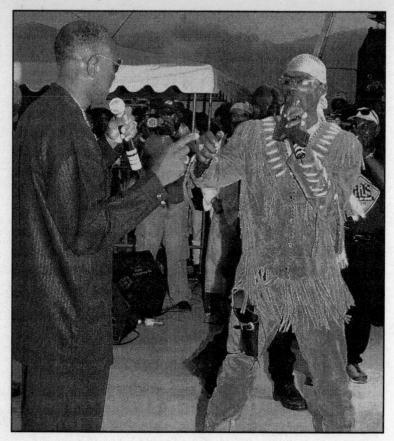

Dancehall DJ Ninja Man brandishing a Glock 9mm pistol (in his left hand) while speaking to Senior Superintendent of Police Reneto Adams (with microphone at left), during his performance at the 2002 "Sting" concert at Jamworld.
He eventually handed over the weapon. Photo: Ian Allen.

Simpleminded evaluations of the verbal violence of Jamaican dance-hall lyrics often fail to take into account the promiscuous genesis of these discourses, instead representing them as unambiguous signs of the congenital pathology of Jamaican popular culture and its creators. Conversely, I argue that *badmanism* is a theatrical pose that has been refined in the complicated socialization processes of Jamaican youths who learn to imitate and adapt the sartorial and ideological "style" of the heroes and villains of imported movies. Cinema remains a relatively cheap form of mass entertainment for the urban poor, though cable television networks increasingly facilitate access to the full range of offerings of the North American film and television industry.

There is, as well, an indigenous tradition of heroic "badness" that has its origins in the rebellious energy of enslaved African people who refused to submit to the whip of bondage. Nanny of the Maroons, for example, is memorialized as having possessed supernatural powers; it is said that she used her bottom to deflect the bullets of British soldiers. Nineteenth-century visionaries like Paul Bogle and Sam Sharpe kept alive the heroic spirit of resistance to the dehumanizing conditions of colonial Jamaica. This militant antislavery, antiestablishment ethos accounts in large measure for much of the ambivalence about "badness" in Jamaican society.

The classic 1972 Jamaican cult film *The Harder They Come* and the much more recent 1999 *Third World Cop* illustrate the indigenization of an imported American culture of "heroism" and gun violence; both films glamorize Hollywood reconstructions of masculinity. These distorted images are greedily imbibed by gullible Jamaican youths searching for role models. In a December 2002 interview with Winford Williams on CVM Television's "On Stage," Ninjaman acknowledged the profound impact that *The Harder They Come* had on him as a vulnerable child. That movie created a taste for the feel of the gun. The DJ persuaded his grandmother to buy him a cowboy suit as a Christmas present and, along with it, he acquired his first set of (toy) guns. On stage at Sting 2002, Ninjaman, dressed in a resplendent gold cowboy costume, dramatically handed over to Senior Superintendent Reneto Adams a Glock 17 pistol, symbolizing his rejection of the culture of gun violence and signaling his support for a gun amnesty that would encourage outlaw gunmen to surrender illegal weapons.

Gleaner columnist Melville Cooke gives a much more sophisticated reading than Boyne's of the theatrical performance of badness in Jamaican culture:

> Ninja Man and Reneto Adams, in their public personae, represent two sides of that much beloved and admired Jamaican personality, the bad man. Ninja Man is the incorrigible, fearless bad man that the supposedly decent citizens of the country would shudder to see at their gate, while SSP Adams is presented as the fearless bad man who stands between the thugs and said supposedly decent citizens.
>
> Make no mistake about it, though, the Ninja and the Saddam are, ultimately, rated for being "real bad man."[4]

Some would argue that SSP Adams is a "*real* bad man" and Ninjaman merely performs badness in his role as the "Original Gold Teeth, Front Teeth, Gun Pon Teeth Don Gorgon." Indeed, in "A Wi Run the Gun Them" Pan Head and Sugar Black, in combination DJ/singer style, assert their own mastery of the discourses of the gun and mockingly claim that Ninjaman is not nearly as bad as the persona he inhabits:

Jamaican:
Ninjaman a talk bout him have fourteen gun
Police hold him the other day, dem never hold him with none
A through him talk too much mek dem lock him down.[5]

English:
Ninjaman claims to have fourteen guns.
The police caught him the other day, but he had not even one gun on him.
It's because he talks too much that they lock him down.

The opening lines of "A Wi Run the Gun Them" level the playing field on which gunmen of various stripes contend: "Respect! All hortical [bonafide] gunman, whether you a police, soldierman or civilian."[6] Furthermore, Pan Head and Sugar Black engage in a lyrical duel/duet in which the DJ's gun salute to badness—a ritual naming of all the weapons he possesses—is counterpointed with the singer's reworking of Dennis Brown's sweet-sounding lovers' rock melody and pointed political lyrics:

> Do you know what it means to have a revolution?
>
> And what it takes to make a solution?
>
> Fighting against the pressure.[7]

Here the gun lyrics that would be dismissed by Boyne as a sign of the gratuitous "violence" of dancehall culture are, in fact, being deployed in the cause of a revolutionary struggle against oppression.

In "How Dancehall Promotes Violence," Boyne attacks the University of the West Indies "intellectuals and other mythmakers" for acknowledging the very connections that the DJs/singers invite us to make:

> They [the mythmakers] give the impression that it is revolutionary violence which the youth are preaching and they even say that Bob Marley and Peter Tosh, who are icons today, preached violence.
>
> It is not the same. There is a difference between an artiste talking about using violence to achieve justice, equal rights and social reform—which the African National Congress (ANC) and other freedom fighters used—and someone promoting anarchistic, nihilistic violence. (Though I am a pacifist myself).[8]

One pacifist's freedom fighter is another's terrorist. And Boyne fails to see the potential for freedom fighting on native soil, instead going far from home for his models of legitimate violence. Somewhat ironically, many African freedom fighters, even Nelson Mandela, acknowledge how much the revolutionary message and music of reggae motivated their own struggle. Dancehall today reincarnates that message in a new body language. But its carnality oftentimes masks its revolutionary political ethos.

Ninjaman's performance of badness and his staged renunciation of it engender similar contradictions. He simultaneously does and does not wish to relinquish his role as *badman*. Having surrendered one gun to SSP Adams, Ninjaman provocatively declared at that Sting 2002 performance that he had another gun that he was keeping for rival DJ Beenie Man. This potentially self-incriminating allegation cannot be simply taken at face value. It illustrates the bravura that is such an essential armament of the braggadocious dancehall performer; it also exemplifies the ongoing verbal clashes between DJs jousting for mastery of the field.

Writing in support of an egalitarian gun amnesty that does not discriminate between the "good" *badman* and the "bad" *badman,* Cooke underscores the rank double standard in Jamaican society that elevates some privileged people above the law and leaves others groveling far below: "We cannot demand that Ninja Man be charged for that particular gun and not question why Bruce Golding was not interrogated about the political violence he said he turned his back on. He must know a lot. We would have to exhume Michael Manley, shake his corpse and ask him about his links to 'Burry Boy' and how he came to be a part of that infamous funeral."[9] Cooke here alludes to the fact that supposedly respectable politicians regularly consort with dons, those alternative authority figures and ambiguous outlaw/heroes of Jamaican popular culture who command massive and dreadful respect. In "Warrior Cause," for example, DJs Elephant Man and Spragga Benz salute a long line of such notorious characters, ascribing to them heroic proportions:

> Well mi [I] come fi [to] big up every warrior
> From di [the] present to di past
> Hail all who know dem [that they] fight for a cause
> ...
> Well some seh [say] dem a bad man

No know di half of it

Don't know a big gill nor a quart of it

Woppy King an Rhygin was di start of it[10]

The metaphor of the gill and the quart (for a little and a lot) exemplifies the inventiveness of the DJs' lyrics: A gill, as defined by the *Oxford English Dictionary* is "[a] measure for liquids, containing one-fourth (or locally, one-half) of a standard pint." A quart is "[a]n English measure of capacity, one-fourth of a gallon, or two pints."

The long list of warriors, with a wonderful assortment of nicknames, includes Feather Mop, Burry Bwoy, Tony Brown, George Flash, Jim Brown, Starky, Dainy, Bucky Marshall, Dudus, Zekes, Ian Mascott, Andrew Phang, Gyasee, Shotta John, Speshie Corn, Claudie Massop, Natty Morgan, Sprat, Sandokhan, Rashi Bull, Cow, Early Bird, Rooster, Chubby Dread, Willy Haggart, George Phang, Tony Welch, Sammy Dread, Randy, and Smile Orange.[11] In this roll call of the rougher than rough and the tougher than tough the DJs include even supposed *badman* lawmen: "Laing an Bigga Ford was di police of it/ . . . / Now Adams come get introduce to it." The somewhat ambivalent DJs also salute potential warriors who renounce the calling:

Big up di youth dem weh [who] steer clear of it

Weh wuda [who would] do nuff [lots of] tings

An dem no hear of it

Weh know wrong from di right an dem aware of it

But dem still no have no coward or no fear of it.

It is not only deprived ghetto youths (whether *badman* or bad cop) who are caught up in the gun culture of Hollywood fantasy and its deadly manifestations in real-life Jamaican society. The Jamaican jazz pianist Monty Alexander, in a rap entitled "Cowboys Talk," nostalgically recalls the cowboy heroes of his childhood, enigmatically linking their apparent demise with the birth of ska: "When I was a *likl* [little] boy I remember we used to go to pictures. Some people say movies. And some people down in Jamaica say 'we going to the flim [*sic*] show.' On a Saturday morning. Matinee. And we used to sit there and watch the greatest cowboy stars on the screen. And I mean Roy Rogers and Gene Autry and all them kind a man dem riding pon the horse. But you know what? Them not riding no more. Is like ghost riders in the ska."[12] Alexander evokes ska instrumental compositions performed by Don Drummond and the Skatalites, such as "Ringo," "Lawless Street," "Guns of Navarone," and "Ska-ta-shot," the titles of which clearly have their genesis in the assimilated culture of the Hollywood Western.

Bob Marley's "I Shot the Sheriff" similarly evokes the seductive gun culture of the Wild West. In a September 1975 interview with musicologist Dermott Hussey, Marley gives an account of the evolution of the song that emphasizes the power of lyrical weaponry: "People fight me, a di more it better fi me. Becau you see when dem fight me, mi can go sit down an meditate of what they fighting me fa and make a song of it. How you think me write all 'Shot di Sheriff' and all dem tune deh? Just the fight weh me a get inna mi own group. Mi ha fi shoot all sheriff."[13]

The symbolic power of the ghetto gunman in *The Harder They Come* is amplified because the *shotta* is also a reggae singer, brilliantly played by the redoubtable Jimmy Cliff. Real-life Rhygin Ivan was no singer. The Perry Henzell/Trevor Rhone adaptation of the Rhygin legend for film distills the essence of urban revolt: the fusion of reggae music and *badmanism,* shaping the sensibility of duppy-conquering ghetto youth like Bob Marley and his dancehall progeny. Rhygin's control of literal/lyrical and symbolic gunfire in *The Harder They Come* is an excellent example of an oral performance tradition in which masking, spectacle, role-play, and sublimation are essential elements. Contemporary Jamaican dancehall music is an organic part of that total theater of Jamaican popular culture and must be read with the same sophistication that other modes of performance demand.

For Ivan, whose sensibility is shaped in part by the fantasy world of film, reggae music is an urgent expression of contemporary social reality. In Richard Thelwell's novelization of *The Harder They Come*, the protagonist muses on the ideological power of reggae: "It seemed to him a sign and a promise, a development he had been waiting for without knowing it. This reggae business—it was the first thing he'd seen that belonged to the youth and to the sufferahs. It was roots music, dread music, their own. It talked about no work, no money, no food, about war an' strife in Babylon, about depression, and lootin' an' shootin', things that were real to him."[14]

"This reggae business" is also a magical enterprise in which poor ghetto youths, identifying with the heroes of Hollywood fantasy, can rise to international fame and fortune. The nom-de-guerre of many DJs, old and new, encodes the film origins of their fantasy personae: Dillinger, Trinity, Ninjaman, Red Dragon, Bandolero. The persistence of this tradition of role-play in contemporary Jamaican dancehall culture makes it difficult sometimes for outsiders to accurately decode local cultural signs. Fusion of the literal and the metaphorical can confuse the issue.

The fact that shooting incidents do occur at some dances, for example, does not invalidate the argument that in many instances gunfire is meant to be purely symbolic. In Jamaican dancehall culture literal gunfire often was used in the past as a dangerous salute in celebration of the verbal skill of the heroic DJ/singer. Over time, this purely ritual gunfire has been replaced by the flashing of cigarette lighters, and, more recently, the brandishing of illuminated cell phones as the preferred signal of the audience's approval of the DJ/singer's lyrics: a symbol of a symbol, the flash of verbal creativity. With the emergence of the "fire man" Rastafari DJs like Sizzla and Capleton, the lighting of the spray from aerosol cans by enthusiastic fans—a decidedly dangerous activity that ought to be banned—creates a whoosh of all-too-real fire to represent the burning flames of the DJ's rhetoric.

In yet another metaphorical turn, the expression "pram, pram!"—a verbal rendering of simulated gunshots—becomes a generic sign of approval of verbal skill beyond the domain of the dancehall. A student at the University of the West Indies, Mona who knows of my interest in the language of the dancehall reported that the minister of her church invoked divine gun shots in his 1993 Easter Sunday sermon: "Jesus Christ is risen, pram pram!"—the dancehall equivalent of "Hosannah in the Highest," I suppose. This is the rhetoric of the "lyrical gun," a turn of phrase deployed by Shabba Ranks in the song "Gun Pon Me:"

> Jamaican:
> When mi talk bout gun it is a lyrical gun
> A lyrical gun dat di people have fun
> Fi gyal jump up an just a rail an bomb
> Niceness deh yah an it can't done[15]

> English:
> When I talk about a gun it's a lyrical gun
> A lyrical gun for the people to have fun
> For women to jump up, go wild, and explode
> Niceness is here and it can't end

The image of the "lyrical gun" vividly illustrates the function of metaphor and role-play in contemporary Jamaican dancehall culture. "Lyrical" is not a word that one would ordinarily use to describe a gun; "lyrical" is the language of poetic introspection, not willful extermination. "Lyrical gun" is a quintessential dancehall term, the language of subversion and subterfuge: mixing things up, turning them inside out and upside down. A lyrical gun is the metaphorical equivalent of a literal gun. Words fly at the speed of bullets and the lyrics of the DJ hit hard. In this context, the word "lyrical," belonging to the domain of verbal play and fantasy, becomes a synonym of "metaphorical."

"Gun Pon Me" is an extended gun salute to Shabba Ranks's own verbal and sexual potency: The lyrical gun clearly assumes phallic proportions. The moving target at which the DJ fires is spellbound female fans from all over the world who respond energetically to the metaphorical shots he discharges, eagerly picking up the spent shells. By contrast, men are discounted as impotent rivals, easily eliminated by the DJ: "If is a bwoy, yes, him get knock out/ An if is a girl she a shock out shock out."[16] [If it's a guy, he'll get knocked out/ And if it's a gal she just struts her stuff.] Shabba militantly declares his mastery of the global field, naming major centers of Jamaican migration: The United Kingdom, Canada, and the city/state, New York, a world unto itself. The DJ's "route" signifies the diasporic sweep of Jamaican popular culture:

Jamaican:

Born as a soldier Shabba Rankin a no scout

An if is di music, run it without a doubt

Control mi control an rule up mi route

Who don't like me tell dem go to hell

Shabba Rankin lyrics have England under spell

Shabba Rankin lyrics ha Jamaica under spell

If is Canada dem know me as well

Inna New York mi career extend

Wi a bus di gun an dem a pick up shell

Wi a di fire di gun an dem a pick up di shell

If is New York everybody can tell

Pamela, Susan, an di one Rachel

If mi don't DJ di world a go rebel

Tell di whole world seh dem under a spell[17]

English:

Born as a soldier Shabba Rankin is no scout

And if it's the music, I run things without a doubt

I'm in full control, and I decide my route

Whoever doesn't like me, tell them to go to hell

Shabba Rankin's lyrics have England under a spell

Shabba Rankin's lyrics have Jamaica under a spell

In Canada they know me as well

In New York my career is on the rise

We're making the gun explode and they're picking up shells

We're firing the gun and they're picking up shells

In New York everybody can tell

Pamela, Susan, and Rachel

If I don't DJ the world is going to rebel

Tell the whole world that they're under a spell

"Gun Pon Me" is a fascinating example of the way in which the lyrics of the DJs traverse ideological spaces, engendering sound clashes between literal and metaphorical discourse. The unsettling first verse reverberates with what seems to be quite literal gunfire. Shabba, who styles himself as "di bad boy fi di girls dem" [the bad boy for the girls] issues a deadly warning to male informers:

Jamaican:

Mi av mi gun pon mi an mi naa tek it out

Why mi naa tek it out? Too much informer deh bout

An mi no waan shoot someone inna dem mouth.

Tongue a jump up an teeth a jump out

Me a bust di gun an dem a pick up shell

Me a fire di gun an dem a pick up di shell

Can't hide mi gun else a guy woulda tell

Way mi gun big, yes, im head woulda swell

Gone go ring mi name like di tongue inna a bell

Mi ha fi slaughter im an done im mada as well.[18]

English:

I have my gun on me and I won't take it out

Why won't I take it out?

There are too many informers about

And I don't want to have to shoot anyone in the mouth.

The tongue is jumping up and teeth are jumping out

I'm making the gun explode and they're picking up the shells

I'm firing the gun and they're picking up the shells

I can't hide my gun or else a guy would tell

My gun is so big, yes, his head would swell

He would go and sound my name abroad

Like a tongue in a bell

I would have to slaughter him

And then finish off his mother as well

It is the later use of the modifier "lyrical" that first signifies the song's ambiguous vacillation between the literal and the metaphorical: "If is Pamela pick up lyrical shell/ If is Susan she pick up di lyrical shell/ An if is Ann-Marie pick up di lyrical shell." [If it's Susan, she's picking up the lyrical shell/ And if it's Ann-Marie she's picking up the lyrical shell.] Shabba's firing of his lyrical gun explosively echoes the identical use of the gun metaphor by old-school reggae artists, for example the Ethiopians in their 1970 song, "Gun Man":

I'm gonna get you down

I'm gonna gun you down

I've got a loaded 45

It's sweet music

I've got a loaded 45

It's soul music

Gun, gun, gun, gunman talk[19]

This conception of music as a "loaded 45"—a lyrical gun—is useful in decoding the rhetoric of gun violence in Jamaican popular music. Understood in its indigenous context, the meaning of the gun lyrics of the reggae singers and dancehall DJs is much less transparent than might initially appear. Thus, for example, an infamous song like Buju Banton's "Boom By-By," which seems on the surface to advocate the literal extermination of homosexuals, may be loaded with multiple meanings—read in the light of Shabba Ranks's "lyrical gun." This I attempted to demonstrate at a December 1992 seminar entitled "Reggae Music as a Business," convened at the Jamaica Conference by Specs-Shang Muzik, Inc. and Sandosa Ltd. in collaboration with the Eagle Merchant Bank, the National Commercial Bank, and the Trafalgar Development Bank. My paper, entitled "Cultural Implications of Marketing Reggae Internationally," focused on the controversial reception of Buju Banton's infamous anti-homosexuality song, whose resonant boom has echoed across continents, generating much public debate.

In my role as cultural critic, I assumed the burden of communal responsibility for the youthful DJ who had put himself at risk by running up his mouth. There are well-defined Caribbean cultural codes that justify this acceptance of communal responsibility. Consider the cultural rules that are at work when the man with mouth is confronted by the man with muscle. The man with mouth bawls out to the community, "Unu hold mi yaa, hold mi yaa, or mi a go kill him" (Hold me back, hold me back, or I'm going to kill him). The man with mouth is depending on the community to protect him because he knows that he dare not attack this formidable enemy he has verbally challenged. So the man with mouth gets to save face. It is the community, not his cowardice, that has restrained him. I concluded my presentation at the seminar with a clear injunction: The DJ must learn to censure herself or himself, otherwise somebody else will do the censuring.

Nevertheless, I ended up in a hostile sound clash with the *Village Voice*. The seminar was reviewed in its "Rockbeat" column on January 19, 1993, with the headline "Africanist Abomination," and my presentation was scathingly indicted:

> By all reports Cooper's speech was the most enthusiastically received of the
> conference. A room full of 300 lawyers, bankers, and music businesspeople
> greeted references to "buttocks" and a Jamaican proverb that goes "Two
> pot cover can't shut" by whistling and banging on tables and gave the
> professor a standing ovation when she concluded. . . . According to Payday
> Records' Patricia Moxey, the Americans stood around afterward saying,
> "Jeez, these people are pretty out there," but saw no way to convey their
> reaction to their hosts. "I don't agree with her views," Moxey told us, "but
> I think she was right about what she was saying about Jamaica—that
> everyone is completely homophobic."

That is decidedly *not* what I was saying. And this reported American
marginalization of Jamaican cultural perspectives as being "pretty out there"
is itself a manifestation of the xenophobia of the *Village Voice,* which had
previously refused to publish my own account of the "Boom By-By" affair.

Indeed, one must immediately raise an admittedly controversial issue
about the function of violent talk in predominantly oral cultures like
Jamaica. Violent, daring talk such as that of the DJ and the rapper can
function as a therapeutic substitute for even more dangerous violent
action. Cathartic talk does not so much incite to violence as it controls
violence in a socially accepted way. This proposition that violent *talk* is
beneficial does perhaps have less currency these days in Jamaica where
relatively easy access to guns seems to have made it increasingly unlikely
that the cultural traditions that once used talk as a beneficial substitute for
physical abuse will be maintained.

Like Rhygin, the DJs often assume a *badman* pose: pure role-play.
Despite Buju Banton's explicit reference to what sounds like frighteningly
literal gunfire—Uzis, and other automatic weapons—"Boom By-By" nevertheless does assume metaphorical significance. Especially if we apply
Shabba's metaphor of the gun as symbolic penis, we can see Buju's use of
the gun in the song in a new light. In the final analysis, it can be read as a

celebration of the vaunted potency of heterosexual men who know how to use their lyrical gun to satisfy their women. After all, in Shabba's "Gun Pon Me" it is Pamela, Susan, and Ann-Marie who pick up the DJ's lyrical shell. The homosexual is safely out of firing range.

Even read in a purely literal-minded way, "Boom By-By" is multilayered. First, the derogatory word *"batty-man"* itself illustrates the use of graphic imagery in Jamaican Creole to express abstraction. The explicit Jamaican word *"batty-man"* encodes a very precise naming of the place to which the sexual propensities of the homosexual are presumed to incline literally. "Batty," the Jamaican Creole word for buttocks, compounded with "man," encodes anal sex. In a synecdochic transfer, the part (the *batty*) comes to stand for the whole (the homosexual). The vivid Jamaican word *batty-man,* unlike the somewhat abstract Greek/Latin/English compound-word "homosexual," illustrates the tendency of speakers of the Jamaican language to employ literal detail in circumstances where speakers of other languages, like English, might use abstraction.

This privileging of the literal to articulate the abstract is not always understood by non-native speakers of Jamaican. Thus, taken out of context, the popular Jamaican Creole declaration, "all batty-man fi dead," may be misunderstood as an unequivocal, literal death-sentence: "all homosexuals must die." Read in its cultural context, this battle cry, which is appropriated by Buju Banton in "Boom By-By," primarily articulates an indictment of the abstraction, homosexuality, which is rendered in typically Jamaican terms as an indictment of the actual homosexual: The person (the homosexual) and the project (homosexuality) are not identical. This distinction is an attempt to explicate how language conveys culture-specific meanings; it is not a duplicitous denial of the fact that the homosexual person is often victimized in Jamaican society.

In some instances homosexuals, like heterosexuals, are victims of domestic violence from their own partners; in other cases they are victims of ritual violence from the homophobic community. This victimization of homosexuals is part of a continuum of violence in Jamaican culture: In much the same way that predial larceny is often punished illegally by angry mobs who take the law into their own hands and lynch the apparently guilty, homosexual behaviors, or even the suspicion of intent, do put the individual at risk—so much so that recently some Jamaican homosexuals have successfully sought asylum in the United Kingdom on grounds of sexual discrimination, though that door has now been firmly closed. In a remarkable sleight of hand, the British government, apparently in response to the increasing numbers of applicants, has unilaterally declared that it is the homosexual "lifestyle," not the individual's life, that is at risk in Jamaica and so those asylum seekers are no longer eligible for automatic protection. Somewhat ironically, the rationale of this politically expedient posture seems quite similar to the Jamaican convention of distinguishing between the homosexual person and practice.

But Robert Carr, a Research Associate in the Centre for Population, Community and Social Change at the University of the West Indies, Mona, Jamaica, documents the extralegal "judgment" that is often meted out to victimized homosexuals in Jamaica:

> Such attacks have a name. They are called "batty judgements." The fact that all of the informants knew what a "judgement" was, although they did not necessarily know each other, attests to the ubiquity of the term. The concept of anything associated with homosexuality brings with it the anathema expressed by adding the term "batty" to the phrase. Thus a group of men was harassed for promoting "batty business" because they had a number of condoms on them that they intended to distribute in promoting safer sex and condom use. "Battyman fi dead" (gay men must die) is a common expression that accompanies the community attacks. In one instance, a large crowd gathered to watch, chanting "battyman, battyman, battyman" while the attack took place. In that instance the man was beaten, kicked, stabbed, had filthy water from the gutter thrown on him by a gang of armed men. This level of brutality was a common thread reported by the informants, although large crowds gathering to watch are less common. The mere fact

that someone is accused of being a "battyman" is sufficient to trigger an attack of such violence.[20]

The biblical term, "judgment," with its Old Testament resonances of immediate fire and brimstone damnation, confirms the fundamentalist Christian genesis of this rampant hatred of homosexual behaviors in Jamaica, in general, and its manifestation in acts of brutality committed by working-class males, in particular. Though the aversion to homosexuality crosses class lines, expressions of physical violence against homosexuals are usually restricted to working-class communities where hierarchies of impoverishment and marginalization are institutionalized. Indeed, class privilege usually insulates middle- and upper-class homosexual males in Jamaica from acts of heterosexist physical violence.

Furthermore, just as prevaricating Christians are taught to "hate the sin and love the sinner," Jamaicans are generally socialized to recognize the fact that anti-homosexuality values are entirely compatible with knowing acceptance of homosexuals within the community. This is a fundamental paradox that illustrates the complexity of the ideological negotiations that are constantly made within the society. Most male homosexuals in Jamaica seem content to remain in the proverbial closet; but the door is wide open. They move comfortably across social borders. Then there are clearly "out" homosexuals who work, for example, as higglers in Jamaican markets and ply their trade with relatively little provocation. Many have mastered the art of "tracing"—ritualized verbal abuse—as a form of protection from the heterophobia of Jamaican society.

In Jamaica, homosexuality is routinely denounced because it is perceived as a marker of difference from the sexual/cultural "norm." Further, many Jamaicans vigorously object to being labeled as "homophobic." Claiming their heterosexuality as "normative," they reject the negative connotations of the "phobia" in homophobia. For them it is homosexuality that is the morbidity—not their culturally legitimated aversion to it.

The credentializing of sexual orientation becomes necessary in a heterophobic society whose political leaders, for example, use the alleged homosexuality of rivals as a deadly weapon. A spectacular example of this legitimating impulse is the surprising public declaration on the radio talk show, the *Breakfast Club,* made by the prime minister of Jamaica, P. J. Patterson, in 2001: "My credentials as a lifelong heterosexual person are impeccable." The opposition Jamaica Labour Party is notorious for attacking Patterson on grounds of color and, more recently, alleged sexual orientation. TOK's popular anti-homosexuality song, "Chi-Chi Man," was used by supporters of the Jamaica Labour Party as a rallying cry during a 2001 by-election campaign.[21] "Chichi man" is current slang for homosexual. The *Dictionary of Jamaican English* defines "chichi" as "the dry-wood termite *Cryptotermes brevis*" and notes that it is "prob[ably] from some African form indicating small size." One wonders if the "chichi man" slang extension of the meaning is intended to represent the homosexual as a diminutive man. Also, since "wood/hood" is a Jamaican Creole metaphor for "penis," "chichi man" could also suggest the vulnerability of the homosexual's manhood to chichi of all kinds.

In addition, "homophobia" in neo-African societies like Jamaica is often conceived as an articulation of an Africanist worldview in which the essential complementary of opposites is affirmed: earth/sky, male/female, etc. There is a popular Jamaican proverb that uses a vivid domestic image to define the "unnaturalness" of homosexuality: "Two pot cover[s] can't shut." The pot (female) and its cover (male) naturally go together. Heterosexual intercourse—the shutting of pot with cover—is idealized as normative. The proverb's clear proscription against the attempt to shut two covers (or, by implication, two pots) can be decoded as an affirmation of Afrocentric norms of sexual propriety.

In my search for an African genesis of the cultural attitudes to homosexuality in Jamaica, I discovered an illuminating paper by Hilary Standing of the School of African and Asian Studies, University of Sussex, England, who in his own words,

Start[s] from the premise that sexual behaviour is socially constructed. That is to say, there are no "natural" sexualities. Rates and forms of expression vary across time and space. The definition adopted incorporates three main elements: (1) specific sexual practices in terms of the forms within which sexual contact occurs; (2) the range and numbers of sexual partners, which leads to a consideration of the social, economic, and political factors which determine or influence the changing of partners; (3) the social meanings of sex in any given context. This includes ideologies of masculinity and femininity, culturally sanctioned modes of sexuality, and sexual expression, and associated forms of control and coercion.[22]

The question, then, for which I was seeking an answer is: What are the social meanings of homosexuality in Sub-Saharan Africa that might have some bearing on Jamaican constructions of sexual identity, given the longevity of other African-derived cultural practices, such as religion, throughout the African diaspora? Standing reports:

Male homosexual practices are also publicly denied and condemned in many African contexts. Their existence in single sex institutions such as the army, prisons, and schools is, however, tacitly acknowledged. What is strongly denied is the concept of homosexuality as a "career," except in some areas of Arab/Islamic influence and where commercialised homosexual services have developed in cities which attract international tourists and businessmen.[23]

He elaborates:

The sexual content of these relationships is variable. Sources in Sudan, central, and southern Africa suggest that sexual contact does not involve anal intercourse but the practice of rubbing the penis between the partner's thighs. However, Shepherd points out that in Mombassa anal intercourse is the norm. This suggests that higher risk practices are distinctively found in areas of sexual tourism and where there are wider, Arabic, European, and American influences.[24]

Standing also argues, "Homosexuality is not necessarily constructed as an exclusive socio-sexual identity as it is in Europe and America."[25] He notes that "Youths involved in such relationships with older men move on at a certain point in their life cycle to relationships with women. Older men have wives as well as young male lovers."[26]

This complex spectrum of socio-sexual identities and behaviors makes it obviously difficult to draw facile comparisons across cultural traditions. But it seems reasonable to conclude from Standing's insistent argument that homosexuality in Sub-Saharan Africa is *not* socially constructed as normative and, indeed, flourishes primarily in areas influenced by the culture of tourism. Thus it may very well be true that two locally produced pot covers won't shut; but all things are possible with the importation of appropriate technology. Biblical prohibitions against homosexuality and Victorian norms of Euro-American morality that have only recently been undermined in our much more liberal times are thus reinforced by Afrocentric proscriptions.

This Jamaicanized Old Testament ideology of (homo)sexual sinfulness has its equivalent expression in other Caribbean countries. There is a Guyanese joke that says "if yu hat fall off yu head in St. James kick it galang." In other words, don't bend down: St. James is the parish in Barbados most noted for homosexuality. Guyana, though geographically South American, is culturally Caribbean. Jamaican literary critic Al Creighton, long-resident there, notes somewhat elliptically in a *Stabroek News* article, "while we can quite easily accept many universal codes of decency, there are acts which might be deemed vulgar by aliens and the uninitiated, which are clean, legitimate factors in the culture of those who practice them."[27] The (hetero)sexual sinfulness of imported dancehall music in the Guyanese context assumes racial overtones as the music becomes identified as a distinctly African, not Indian, form.

In Barbados, heterosexual resistance to homosexuality and especially bisexuality is evident, for example, in a vociferous newspaper column written by "Lick Mout Lou" [gossiping Lou] who, in a letter to a friend, Nesta, lashes out in the Barbadian vernacular against "de bunch o' nasty bisexual men we got 'bout hey [dat] is de ones mainly responsible fuh de spread o' Aids."[28] She elaborates:

> I hear de figure is 60 per cent bisexuals 'mong de male population.
>
> So you would onderstan' hummuch women boun' to get infeck after dem wutliss [worthless] men dat does drive 'bout at night pickin' up male prostitutes get back home to got sex wid duh women. 'Nough so-call decent, Christian-minded wives dat does be home cookin' an' sewin' an' waitin' fuh duh [for their] husbands gine [are going to] be Aids victims, you wait an' see.
>
> I gine tell yuh de troot [truth], Ness—Buhbayduss in 1992 en nuh diff'rent from Sodom an' Gomorrah. . . . I only hope dat wid all de wutlissness dat gine on, de wife swappin an' de blue movies an' de t'ings dat gine on at a certain club when de night come, dat de Mighty Jehovah don' wipe de islan' off de map wid some catastrophe, nuh joke![29]

In Barbados, imported Jamaican dancehall music and local varieties do reinforce anti-homosexuality norms of propriety even while simultaneously attracting abuse by defying traditional norms of heterosexual propriety. This is a fascinating paradox.

The ambiguous placement of homosexuals in Jamaican society is clearly exemplified in the case of the local reception of "Boom By-By." There was no immediate public outcry against the song from homosexuals in Jamaica, largely because at the time there was no public lobby group. Since then JFLAG (the Jamaican Forum for Lesbians, All-Sexuals and Gays) has emerged as the standard bearer of a more liberal sexual politics around matters of homosexuality. For conservative Jamaicans, the acronym JFLAG is itself somewhat of a red flag fanning the flames of heterophobia. The *Star* of Monday November 2, 1992, promised that prominent local homosexuals were planning to organize to fight the threat of violence against homosexuals, but no prominent spokesman was actually named. The impetus to publicly protest in Jamaica the heterophobia of "Boom By-By" seems to have come from Europe and North America, where groups like the Gay & Lesbian Alliance Against Defamation (GLAAD) gladly turned the song into a cause (in)célèbre.

Several weeks after the international protest against "Boom By-By" had been launched, rumors began to circulate in Jamaica that local homosexuals were going to hold a protest march in Kingston that would converge in Half-Way-Tree Square/Mandela Park. The talk was greeted with disbelief, though on the day of the rumored march, men of all social classes gathered in the square, armed with a range of implements—sticks, stones, machetes—apparently to defend their collective heterosexual honor, Old Testament style. The march did not take place. The furor surrounding the event provided a melodramatic opportunity for Jamaican society to articulate both its resistance to and its tolerance of homosexuality. Numerous callers on various talk shows aired their opinions in defense of or attack on the homosexual's right to freedom of expression. Somewhat paradoxically, this public debate is the positive spin-off from Buju's controversial song. Jamaican society has been forced to confront openly the taboo subject of homosexuality within our community. Significantly, it is the popular forms of cultural expression like dancehall lyrics that are generating open debate.

The politics of representation are complicated: It would appear that homosexuals in Jamaica themselves accept the social contract, proverbially expressed, "where ignorance is bliss, 'tis folly to be wise." Coming out leaves no room for blissful ignorance of one's sexual preference. It allows no uncontested space for role-play. Migration from the closed, heterophobic world of Jamaican society does facilitate less ambiguous modes of self-representation. For example, it is rumored in Jamaica that the lyrics of "Boom By-By" were translated for GLAAD by a migrant Jamaican homosexual living in New York. This collaboration of North American and

Jamaican homosexuals marks a new stage of politicization of consciousness outside of, and within, Jamaica around issues of heterophobia.[30]

Furthermore, in the U.S. export market, where the multivalent Jamaican cultural terms of reference are not clearly understood, indigenous
cultural texts like Buju Banton's "Boom By-By" can be taken all too
literally out of context. For example, Ransdell Pierson reports in an article
headlined "'Kill Gays' Hit Song Stirs Fury":

> Two organizations, the Gay & Lesbian Alliance Against Defamation and
> Gay Men of African Descent, insisted yesterday they weren't trying to
> censor the song from the airwaves.
>
> But they also insisted that if radio stations are callous enough to
> broadcast it, they should help prevent actual bloodshed by running public-
> service announcements denouncing anti-gay violence.
>
> "Without such announcements, these stations are promoting the
> message that young people should attack lesbians and gay men," said
> Donald Suggs, a GLAAD spokesman.[31]

It is instructive to note that in Jamaica, where strict censorship laws
apply, provocative songs like "Boom By-By" are not broadcast on the
public media. This fact illustrates a major problem with the indiscriminate
exporting of Jamaican popular culture. The decontextualized export
product is transmitted with no reference to its culture-specific meanings.
In this process, norms of public propriety in Jamaica are often violated.
Whereas "Boom By-By" received wide air play in North America, local
censorship practices in Jamaica control the spread of potentially offensive
songs on the public airwaves. Admittedly, the openness of the open-air
dancehall in Jamaica makes the distinction between public and private
airwaves somewhat academic. Uncensored sound systems do indeed
facilitate public exposure of officially censored music. Nevertheless, the
official censors scrupulously maintain the illusion of public propriety.

In a remarkable 2002 case, the BBC World Service was reprimanded by the Broadcasting Commission of Jamaica for airing a sample of "Boom By-By" in a program documenting the plight of Jamaican homosexuals seeking asylum in the United Kingdom. A press release from the Commission, dated November 25, 2002, summarizes the matter:

BBC Violation

The Commission found that the British Broadcasting Corporation (BBC), holder of a special license permitting relay of its World Service programming on Jamaican airwaves, committed breaches of the Regulations during a transmission on October 28, 2002.

The BBC contravened Regulation 30(d) and (l) when it included documentary clips of a song by local artiste Buju Banton containing an indecent colloquialism used to describe homosexual men and lyrics that explicitly supported violence against this group. Extracts of "Boom Bye Bye" were played during the programme, "Outlook", which was aired at 2:00 p.m. local time.

The BBC has been directed to apologise to its Jamaican audience within fourteen days.[32]

Somewhat ironically, in this instance, the local Broadcasting Commission's well-intentioned act of censorship functions, in effect, to repress the very critique of "indecent" cultural values that is at the heart of its mission. Strict attention to the letter of the law thus violates its spirit. The BBC's apology does concede that an error of editorial judgment may have been made on its part; but it also seems to intimate that the Jamaican Broadcasting Commission's own judgment may not have been fine enough:

On 28th October, the BBC's Outlook programme broadcast a report on homophobia in Jamaica which used extracts of the song "Boom Bye Bye." The Broadcasting Commission of Jamaica found that the use of the song was in breach of their broadcasting regulations related to the transmission of content which might offend against good taste, decency or public morality. Editorial decisions about good taste and decency often involve fine judgements. The decision to add the song to the report was made after very careful consideration at the BBC. But despite that, and in view of the Broadcasting Commission's findings, the BBC would like to apologise to any listeners who were offended by our use of the song.[33]

Cordell Green, chairman of the Broadcasting Commission of Jamaica, observes in e-mail correspondence with me, "the regulations have since been qualified by the Children's Code for Programming which came into force on January 13, 2003. The Code recognises that otherwise problematic material may be found acceptable for broadcast if used for educational or journalistic purposes."[34]

The fate of Buju's "Boom By-By" in the *outernational* market, particularly in the United States and United Kingdom, where highly politicized groups of male and female homosexuals wield substantial power, is a classic test case of the degree to which local Jamaican cultural values can be exported without censure into a foreign market. It also raises the issue of language in DJ culture, and the separation of aesthetic and ideological issues that can arise in the exporting of Jamaican music. Non-Jamaicans can appreciate the aesthetically appealing noises of the music without understanding the words. Once they understand the words, they may not be able to accept the cultural message in the music. They may reject the music altogether. How should the reggae artist respond to this ideological/marketing problem? Adapt the message to suit the export market, sacrificing authenticity for airplay? Should the artist do one kind of song for the local market and another for export? Or should the reggae artist risk censorship in order to maintain the cultural integrity of the Jamaican worldview?

More complex legal and commercial issues arise as a result of the mode of production of the predominantly oral "text." The exporting of reggae music raises the challenging question of multiple rights: copyright, language rights and literacy rights, particularly in an export market where the protection of rights is accomplished in the discourse of writing. Consider for example the case of the publication of an unauthorized English translation of "Boom By-By" that appeared as "Boom Bye-Bye" in the Pierson article. The translation, supplied by GLAAD, can be quite fairly described as biased against Buju. Translation is clearly an ideological issue. For instance, what looks like a minor matter, the addition of an "e" to "By," reinforces the sinister qualities of the song—saying permanent good-bye, a deadly ironic farewell. In his *Village Voice* exposé on "Batty Boys in Babylon," Trinidadian journalist Peter Noel works the idea of good-bye to a tearful conclusion. Having explained to a young relative, "This song is about killing your uncle," he quotes the child as saying "Sorry, uncle. Bye bye, Buju."[35]

In addition, there are several instances of mistranslation. For example, "homeboy" is not an accurate translation of "rudeboy." The Jamaican word connotes a whole history of resistance that has been legitimized in the evolution of Jamaican popular music. The classic Jamaican movie *The Harder They Come,* for example, gives us the ideological justification of the making of a rudeboy. The (mis)translation of "rude" boy as "home" boy thus elides the specificity of the history of working-class resistance in urban Jamaica. The African American word "homeboy"—meaning, approximately, the Jamaican "yardie"—does not have the precise cultural authority that would legitimate the righteous rudeboy posture that Buju assumes in the opening frame of "Boom By-By." The mistranslation "homeboy" dislocates Buju's imported DJ aesthetics and places his song in the already prejudiced context of African American rap. The DJ is forced to take the rap.

Indeed, Pierson's article concludes by implying an exact parallel between "Boom By-By" and Ice-T's "Cop Killer." A fair cross-cultural, Afrocentric comparison can be made, but not an exact parallel drawn, if you know the Jamaican context of Buju's song. The DJ's rudeboy lyrics, decontextualized, assume all the negative associations that stigmatized rap is forced to bear in the delegitimizing discourse of dominating, mono-cultural white American political correctness. The element of metaphor and role-play that is such a crucial aspect of Jamaican popular culture (and rap) is undermined in Pierson's literal-minded reading of the DJ's lyrics: "This past summer, rapper Ice-T triggered a major controversy with his song 'Cop Killer,' whose lyrics encouraged murdering police officers. He eventually removed it from his album *Body Count,* produced by Warner Records."[36]

The mistranslated, sadomasochistic lines, "Girls bend over and take your dick/ And even if it really hurts/ She still won't refuse," are equally problematic. The *New York Post* front-page headline defines Buju's song as "Hate Music." These mistranslated lines extend the "hate" from homosexuals to women. The original Jamaican lines are "Gyal bend down back way an accept di peg/ An if it really hot she still naa go fleg." I propose an alternative translation: "The woman bends down backways and accepts the peg/ And if it's really hot she still won't get tired."[37] In Jamaican Creole, "it hat" is ambiguous: both, "it hurts" and "it is hot." Is "hot" exclusively "hurt," as it is translated here by GLAAD? Or does Buju's "hot" mean not so much the inflicting of pain as the celebrating of the acrobatic skill of "hot" women who know how to bend down backways to receive a certain kind of pleasurable heat? The women's backward bending to deliver her front is clearly being contrasted with the back entrance that the *batty-man* is forced to use. The original "peg" is also much more allusive than "dick."

A particularly problematic mistranslation is the substitution of "firewood" for the original "tyre wheel" in the line "Burn him like old firewood." The graphic burning tire wheel image suggests the necklacing of traitors in South Africa. Add to this Chalice's song "P.W. Botha is a batty-man," and Shabba Ranks's dismissal (on a BBC interview) of charges of "slackness" with the retort that apartheid is slackness; one begins to see a pattern of ideological convergence in which both homosexuality and racism are constructed in dancehall culture as equally illegitimate.

To Jamaican ears Buju Banton's "Boom By-By" is as much about "the sweetness between women's legs" as it is an indictment of homosexuality. Here, perhaps, we see in the diaspora remnants of West African female fertility cults in which the celebration of female sexuality is ritualized. The representation of woman in dancehall culture as powerful sexual agents is an affirmation of the capacity of the female body to generate submissive respect, however much male devotees may "mask" this respect in the apparently abusive catalog of glorified female body parts. The same Buju Banton in yet another controversial song expresses his devotion to an admired female in terms that evoke rapacious gun violence: He has to have the woman's body even if it is at gunpoint. Here the line between lyrical and literal gun is dangerously blurred:

> Hear weh [what] me tell di girl seh if unu look good!
>
> Hear weh me tell her seh!
>
> Gyal me serious
>
> Mi ha fi [I have to] get yu tonight
>
> Even by gun point[38]

Imported western feminist notions of "misogynist" Jamaican dancehall culture may be constituted as yet another example of heterophobia— the devaluation of misunderstood local cultural traditions. Consider, for example, the intersection of spirituality and carnality in traditional John Canoe/jonkunnu festivities in Jamaica. The alternate spellings signify the English/West African etymologies of the word. "John Canoe" is defined in the *DJE* as "[t]he leader and chief dancer of a troop of negro dancers. He wears an elaborate horned mask or head-dress, which, by the end of the 18th and early 19th cents, had developed into or been replaced by the representation of an estate house, houseboat, or the like (never a canoe). The celebration takes place during the Christmas holidays, the John Canoe leading the other masqueraders in procession singing and dancing, with drums and noisy 'music', and asking for contributions from bystanders and householders." Historian John Rashford notes, "objects named 'John' are often associated in Jamaica with the world of spirits," thus underscoring the African genesis of what now appears to be secularized religious practices transformed into entertainment in the annual jonkunnu ritual celebration.[39]

Furthermore, despite the recent attempts to revive traditional jonkunnu masquerading as part of the "cultural heritage" of Jamaica, these festivities were actually banned in the early twentieth century because of their potential for disturbing the peace. This punitive control of African Caribbean popular culture foreshadows the current attempts to repress the rebellious energy of the dancehall. The representation of the traditional male jonkunnu masquerader, with his phallic sword and surrounded by admiring females, that is given by the plantocratic historian Edward Long is remarkably similar to the contemporary image of the DJ surrounded by predominantly female fans: "carrying a wooden sword in his hand, [he] is followed with a numerous crowd of drunken women, who refresh him frequently with a sup of aniseed-water whilst he dances at every door, bellowing out *John Connu!* with great vehemence."[40]

An important segment of the implied dancehall audience in Buju's song, as in Shabba Ranks's "Gun Pon Me," is not gun-toting homophobic men but heterosexual women who have a vested interest in the DJ's peg. The more homosexuals there are, the fewer "real" men available to service the agile women: "Happy an yu love it/ yu fi ju-just/ boom by-by." [If you're happy and you love it/ You should just/ boom by-by.] The "boom by-by" here clearly becomes a gun salute to heterosexuality itself, rather than the inciting to violence against homosexuals. Even if we do allow that Buju's song may indeed affirm the authority of violence as a means of social control, we need to recognize that delegitimized ghetto gun violence is the underground equivalent of our official systems of enforced control. The ghetto gun salute becomes the parodic "grassroots" equivalent of the "twenty-one gun salute" that is given to national heroes and thus legitimated by the state. The misguided heroism of ghetto gunmen that manifests itself in elaborate role-play ought to be channeled into more legitimate modes of expression.

Buju Banton's "Mr Nine," from his 2003 CD *Friends for Life,* exemplifies both the complexity of the metaphor of the lyrical gun in Jamaican dancehall culture and the DJ's own ideological development.[41] Gone is the old rhetoric of "Boom By-By," with its explicit condemnation of homosexuality in the language of the lyrical gun. Instead, as in Buju's "Murderer," it is the culture of the gun itself that is under lyrical fire: "I tell unu, all man are created equal/ But behind the trigger it's a different sequel."[42] Cecil Gutzmore gives a compelling reading of this enigmatic couplet:

> . . . "sequel" has a number of meanings appropriate to Buju's context, including "issue, result, upshot." There is even a mediaeval/feudal meaning that has very much to do with the social inequality of lord and villein. And buried within this couplet is the suggestion of a play upon the contradictory notions of equality and inequality. The gun, especially the six-shooter of all those Westerns watched in the land of *The Harder They Come* and which still inhabit the Jamaican popular imagination, is known as the equalizer. This deadly equalizer is the face-to-face eliminator of all those inequalities that developed between that distant, original God-act which created all persons equal and now, when some are so much more equal than others. But the equalizer also imposes a stark inequality between its holder and s/he who is made to stare down its barrel/nozzle.[43]

In "Mr Nine," Buju conjures up a surreal scenario in which personified guns, contesting for the control of territory, critique each other's behavior and simultaneously bewail the battles that are being fought by youths in their name. It is as if the big guns themselves have now assumed control of both the society and their own policing—the authority having slipped from human hands. In a parodic council of elders, Mr Nine and Mr 45 lament the deplorable behavior of M16 and Magnum who are totally out of control. The jumpy German Luger and the AK are responsible for the deaths of many youth. The Ar15 is used to terrorize residents of small communities. The MAC11 keeps on making trouble and the 38 is jealous of the GLOCK's popularity. The 380MATIC thinks of himself as a big shot and the M1 insists on being treated with dignity. The HK Bomber reigns supreme in some communities.[44]

In "Mr Nine," there is a seeming sound clash between what could be heard as a celebratory roll call of these many guns and the DJ's indictment of the culture of gun violence in Jamaica. Buju Banton documents a number of instances in which guns are constantly employed, recalling both legendary moments in the life of particular brands, such as the 303 used to kill Kennedy, as well as the more mundane circumstances in which guns like the "pumprifle," for example, are selected to protect Brinks' employees. Naming the country of origin of some of these guns—Germany and Israel, for example—Buju thus implicates the manufacturers in the capitalist reproduction of international violence.

Not surprisingly, the DJ gestures toward the culture of the Hollywood western recalling that John Wayne's weapon of choice was a Smith and Weston. The romanticization of gun violence and the celebration of badness, as in the globalized U.S. film industry, are signaled in the salute to the Tommy, Gatlin, SMG and Remington. In the silences between the firing of the guns, Buju Banton intersperses warnings to the Jamaican people to emancipate ourselves from the tyranny of the gun and the splitting of justice which these weapons engender. As in his classic lament, "Murderer," the DJ explicitly denounces the murderous gun culture with its paradoxical death-in-life ethos, observing that the authority of the gun and the destructive cycle of violence it perpetuates are perniciously reaffirmed when one yields to the temptation to valorize, as the sustainer of life, an instrument of death.

The function of metaphor and role-play in Caribbean popular culture is not always fully understood within and outside the indigenous context. Thus, the lyrics of Jamaica's dancehall DJs, taken all too literally, have increasingly come under attack at home and abroad. Somewhat paradoxically, in the battle of symbolic lyrics versus real political clout, it is the DJ himself who must often run for cover. For example, powerful organizations of homosexuals in the North Atlantic like GLAAD seem to be playing the role of imperial overlords in the cultural arena. Their heterophobic politics make little allowance for culture-specific definitions of norms of appropriate sexual behavior. The homogenizing imperative of global political correctness effaces cultural difference in a new imperialism of "liberal" ideology.

Even more important, perhaps, is the possibility that culture-specific discursive strategies that function to "mask" meaning may, in practice, not be acknowledged as legitimate. There is the presumption of a "universal" (English) language of transparent meaning. The cultural arrogance of the new politically correct liberals is thus no different in kind from the cultural arrogance of old world imperialists who knew that Europe was the center of the world and "far-out" territories were just waiting to be discovered. Xenophobia is no less a phobia than homophobia. But all phobias are not created equal. Some (hetero)phobias are more politically correct than others.

The international marketing of reggae is raising fundamental questions about cultural identity, cultural autonomy, and the right to cultural difference. On the issue of sexual preference, Jamaican society is itself slowly moving in the direction of giving visible cultural space to homosexuals. However, given the historical context of a dislocating politics of Euro-American imperialism in the region, "hard-core" Jamaican cultural nationalists are likely to resist any reexamination of indigenous values that is perceived as imposed on them by their imperial neighbor in the North. This heterophobic, neoimperialist offensive may backfire. For example, Jamaican journalist Michael Conally, in a story on "Boom By-By" headlined "Defen' it," observes that "now that Buju is signed to Mercury/Polygram, a major record company, in order not to hurt potential sales, a bit of PR to smooth out the edges might help. However, this smoothing out is causing sections of the grass roots [*sic*] fans to be questioning his sexual preference. It is a well known fact, they charge, that it is 'pure batty man and coke heads weh control the top end of the music business.'"[45] As Buju Banton's "Mr Nine" so lucidly illustrates, with its ambivalent glorification and renunciation of the gun culture in Jamaica, the battle for the fundamental transformation of Jamaican society must first be fought and won on native soil.

SIX

"More Fire"

Chanting Down Babylon
from Bob Marley to Capleton

> So if a fire mek i bun
>
> An if a blood mek i run
>
> Rasta deh pon top
>
> Can't you see?
>
> So you can't predict the flop
>
> Gotta lightning, thunder, brimstone an fire, fire
>
> Lightning, thunder, brrrr brimstone an fire
>
> Oh ya, fire, oh ya
>
> Kill, cramp an paralyze
>
> All weak-heart conception
>
> Wipe dem out of creation, yeah!

These incendiary lyrics, however contemporary they may sound, are not the words of Sizzla, Anthony B, Capleton, or any of the "fire bun" Bobo Dreads whose metaphors inflame today's dancehall consciousness. The rhetoric is vintage Bob Marley: "Revolution," from the 1974 *Natty Dread* album. These days it is easy to forget the blood-and-fire, lightning-thunder-and-brimstone Bob Marley. The revolutionary Tuff Gong Rastaman has been commodified and repackaged as our "One Love" apologist for the Jamaican tourist industry. But it is not fair to blame the Jamaica Tourist Board entirely for the metamorphosis. Many factors account for the up-marketing of Marley's image. First of all, dead men sing no songs. Rereleases, yes, but no new songs. And they cannot protest against the politics of appropriation. If Marley were alive today, he probably would be singing the very same range of songs as he did before he was cut down prematurely—songs chanting down Babylon in its many guises, and songs of love and reconciliation.

But the passage of time often produces selective memory in both individual and national consciousness. So in some quarters, Bob Marley is now hallowed, set up on a pedestal as the epitome of pacifist reggae consciousness. His own grounding in Kingston's concrete jungle and his militant songs of social protest are conveniently forgotten. From that height of near divinity he is routinely summoned to cast down judgment on the generation of vipers that are the contemporary dancehall DJs. Indeed, any attempt to dare to suggest continuities between the work of Bob Marley and that of the DJs is seen as sacrilegious. Entertainment columnist Balford Henry reports the contempt that many old school musicians feel for the up-and-coming DJs:

> One of the problems eating at the root of our music, [sic] is the fact that so many of the important players are so subjective in their outlook. They think that good music either started or ended with their generation.
>
> This sort of thinking has created divisions in the industry. For example, the more experienced musicians, whose guidance the young need to overcome the drawbacks in the music, refuse to work with the youth and distance th[e]mselves from their music, often referring to it in terms like "bup bup" or "Boogooyaga."[1]

The derisory, onomatopoeic "bup bup" evokes the potent beats of the DJs *riddims*. According to the *Dictionary of Jamaican English, buguyaga* is "a word of mixed elements, evid[ently] compounded in Jamaica—cf [confer, compare] BUBU, BUGABOO, BUGO-BUGO for the notion of something ugly, repulsive, unclean, and Ewe *yaka, yakayaka,* disorderly, confused, untidy, slovenly; cf also Hausa *buguzunzumi,* a big fat untidy person." One of the meanings of *buguyaga* given in the dictionary is particularly relevant to contemporary Jamaican dancehall culture: "A dance of some kind—perhaps a low-class or indecent one? Cf buru."

The uncertainty of meaning signaled by the dictionary's cautious question mark is undermined when one does compare the meaning of "buru," which, despite its "folk" pedigree, bears all the marks of the class snobbery that is applied to contemporary dancehall culture: "1. a type of dancing, sometimes vulgar, or an occasion upon which there is such dancing. Spec[ifically] funeral-celebration dancing. . . . 2. A place where wild or indecent dancing is done. . . . 3. A type of music—esp drumming— such as is used for buru dancing; also a drum and a group of musicians who play buru dance music. . . . 4. A cult similar to kumuna, [*sic*] in which wild dancing to drums is a prominent feature."

For that latter definition, the dictionary cites a 1958 quotation from the linguist David DeCamp, "/buru/ some sort of semi-religious order . . . most or all adherents are ex-convicts. They beat kumina drums and use the kumina songs and dances but apparently without any real belief in it." DeCamp's contemptuous allusion to "ex-convicts," compounded with his skepticism about their religious conviction, clearly locates this tradition of "vulgar" buru dancing within the domain of transgressive outsiderness.

This is exactly how today's DJs are viewed by many cultural purists: as a criminal aberration. Indeed, Marley's sacred lyrical epistles to the Jamaicans are sullied in the perverse act of attempting to establish a line of descent from these master texts to contemporary Jamaican popular "music." Descent is definitely a matter of going several steps down the musical scale; and, indeed, the very notion of "descent" is seen as indecent. But, surely, without detracting from the distinctiveness of Bob

Marley's sensibility and the profundity of his contribution to Jamaican and world culture, it must be appropriate to acknowledge the social, political, economic, and other conditions in Jamaica that combined to create his not-so-unique circumstances, against which he rebelled with such passion. These dehumanizing conditions remain potent social forces shaping the consciousness of a new generation of artists and constitute for them sources of inspiration, creativity, as well as despair.

Literal genealogy would suggest that it is to Bob Marley's biological children that one ought to look to find the Marley musical legacy in its purest form. And there is ample evidence that they have taken up the mantle. But it would be naive to expect that they will sing exactly the same kind of songs that their father composed. To the best of my knowledge, Bob Marley's progeny are all children of relative privilege—material privilege. They have not lived the exact circumstances of his fabled life: rural upbringing with a religious mother; urban drift into the concrete jungle of Kingston; brief migration to the United States to do factory work; return to yard roots; unprecedented rise to international superstardom. Their lives are far more ordinary. Somewhat ironically, Bob Marley's lowly origins in material, not spiritual, impoverishment enriched his vision of who he could become. Necessity really is the mother of invention. And each generation sings the songs of its own invention; the necessities may be different, but the capacity for invention remains constant.

Indeed, Bob Marley's ideological heirs are far more likely to originate in the new generation of sufferers who have not yet managed to travel the social distance from Trench Town to Hope Road and up into the hills of privilege. And they are multitudinous. Suffering is the generic condition of the impoverished masses of the Jamaican people, most of whom, nevertheless, ambitiously strive to improve their circumstances. In the words of Bounty Killer:

Jamaican:
Mama she a sufferah

Papa im a sufferah

Can't mek mi children grow up turn sufferah.[2]

English:

Mama is a sufferer

Papa is a sufferer

I can't allow my children to grow up and become sufferers.

Skill at creating and performing lyrics about their own reality will give a few of this generation some access to material prosperity. But most live with a pervasive sense of alienation from Babylon and its culture of scarce benefits and spoils. In failing to remember Bob Marley's own fiery chanting down of Babylon, Jamaican society does him, and his potential beneficiaries, a grave injustice. Cut off unnaturally from the contemporary generation of DJ chanters, Marley is made inaccessible to them as a credible role model of social protest.

Marley's biological children themselves understand the need to bridge the ideological and rhythmic divide between their father's generation and their own. They have experimented with his music, cutting and mixing it with dancehall, rap, and R&B, thus making it over for consumption by their contemporaries. *Chant Down Babylon,* produced by Stephen Marley, exemplifies this innovative trend. In a *Rhythm* magazine cover story, music journalist Patricia Meschino highlights the problematic outcome, for some purists, of that experiment: "Amid crackling simulated gunfire, Gang Starr's Guru delivers grim ghetto realities on 'Johnny Was' (from Bob's 1973 album *Burnin'*). Busta Rhymes' well-placed raps transform the sacred 'Rasta Man Chant' into a [*sic*] urban anthem, and Lauryn Hill turns 'Turn Your Lights Down Low' (from 1977's *Kaya*) into a contemporary soul classic. But though *Chant Down Babylon* has received favorable reviews and spent months on *Billboard*'s R&B chart, the album has caused consternation among music fans who believe the reggae master's work shouldn't be tampered with."[3]

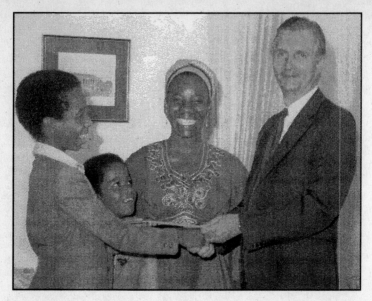

Prime Minister Edward Seaga (right), presents a letter informing Jamaica's Reggae superstar Bob Marley of the honor Order of Merit being conferred on him by the Government and people of Jamaica to David Marley, son of Bob at Jamaica House in April 1981. Mrs. Rita Marley, wife of Bob, and Steve, their younger son, show their appreciation with smiles. Photo: *Gleaner* Archives, 1981.

In response, Stephen Marley is philosophical: "Controversy has been around from ever since the time my father did all those love songs and songs like 'Punky Reggae Party.'" He says, "People would say, 'How he talk about punk?'. . . "My father was not stagnant in music; he was ahead of the time because of the elements he used."[4] Stephen elaborates:

> The people that say the music shouldn't be touched is those that know that music and get it. . . . But all them people that listen to Tupac and the gangsta rap, them no get it. The '70s, that culture and that time, was a very a revolutionary essence, which a lot of older people had the opportunity to grasp and be affected by. It's different now, but back in that time, it changed them life, because they never hear nothing like that before. Now you have a whole heap of different things to show to the youth today; them get more of a thug mentality. But we are

the living testimony of my father, and what you don't know, me can tell you. And

I can tell you in my heart, my father woulda dig this record.[5]

The compelling argument in favor of this experimental album is the "living testimony" of Stephen himself: "This thing is about change; it's about building bridges, bringing people together. It's not about separating. Many people come to me and say, 'My kids are singing [Bob Marley songs] now.' That makes me smile."[6]

The full spectrum of the Marley repertoire is heard on *Chant Down Babylon*. Conversely, in facile revisionist readings of Bob Marley's work, it is the singular "One Love" message that is projected both inside and outside of Jamaica as the sum total of the Gong's philosophy. Even though the ideal of universal love is indeed a noble sentiment (and it is good that "One Love" was dubbed "Song of the Century" by the BBC), one cannot glibly rewrite history. Quite early in his career, Bob Marley *sighted* universal injustice as a destructive force that needed to be chanted down in order for "One Love" to become a real possibility. So he fought a full-scale lyrical war against the ubiquitous forces of evil.

We hear the sounds of war, too, in the speech of His Imperial Majesty Emperor Haile Selassie I delivered in California on February 28, 1968, and which Bob Marley amplified so potently in his commanding performance of the spoken text, the musical score of which was written by Allan Cole and Carlton Barrett (if the skimpy liner notes are accurate):

Until the philosophy which hold one race superior

And another inferior

Is finally and permanently discredited and abandoned

Everywhere is war[7]

Bob Marley was consumed with a passion for social, political, and economic transformation of unjust systems of oppression. But even when it is acknowledged that he did chant down/burn down Babylon, it is his difference from, not his kinship with, contemporary chanters that is emphasized by the revisionists. Marley is celebrated as a master of non-threatening metaphor; the contemporary DJs are dismissed as literal-minded arsonists.

An excellent example of this simplistic rhetoric appears in a *Los Angeles Times* article on the macabre murders committed in the Catholic cathedral in St. Lucia in December 2000 in the name of Rastafari. Under the heading, "Attack Points to 'Lethal' Mix of Religion, Rebellion, Drugs"—a paraphrase of a statement made by Prime Minister Kenny Anthony—reporter Mark Fineman writes an inflammatory article that demonizes Rastafari. Beneath a mountain of innuendo about Rastafari and reggae lies buried one solitary reference to the obvious craziness of the murderers: "Non-Rastafarians privately have voiced their own fears that the violence on the last day of the millennium was not, as police and commentators say, an apparently isolated attack by deranged individuals."[8]

As reported by Fineman, Prime Minister Anthony clearly understands the destabilizing social and economic forces that impact on alienated youth in St. Lucia and the wider Caribbean: "The Caribbean is going through a very, very, very difficult period. We are all troubled, troubled because we are witnessing the increasing marginalization of young males at an uncontrollable rate. We are troubled by rising poverty and crime. And we are troubled by an increasingly unfriendly global [economic] environment."[9] Nevertheless, despite this insight into the local consequences of the disempowering politics of globalization that can make fragile individuals implode, it is the lyrics of DJs like Sizzla that supposedly account far more fully for lunatic behavior. The psychological imbalance of deranged murderers who do not have the good sense to distinguish between literal and metaphorical fire is downplayed:

> "In a lot of Sizzler's songs you hear things like 'Burn down Babylon; Burn down the Vatican; Burn down the pope'" said Peter "Ras Ipa" Isaac, who

heads St Lucia's Imperial Ethiopian World Federation and is among the Rastafarians' old guard here—a group that is deeply concerned about the religion's younger members and its future direction.

"It's not literal," Isaac said. "But in the young minds, like these two guys perhaps, maybe they are influenced in a literal way by these lyrics."[10]

Similarly, Monsignor Theophilus Joseph, administrator of the ill-fated cathedral, observes: "There's a new era—a new kind of protest song that is more violent than the Bob Marley era. It's a very violent message that no doubt is influenced by the American negative rap."[11] Yet another scapegoat, rap. And for the *L.A. Times* journalist, not just the monsignor, the music of the DJs must take the singular blame for the murder in the cathedral: "For much of this young generation, the religion [Rastafari] is also grounded in music. The lyrics have evolved from reggae Rasta star Bob Marley's 'One Love' and his metaphoric references to 'bombing the church' to the incendiary incantations of more recent Jamaican Rastafarian stars such as Sizzler."[12] I am surprised that Fineman used the word "evolved," not "devolved." Be that as it may, it is instructive that, yet again, Bob Marley's supposedly innocuous "metaphoric references" are contrasted with Sizzla's "incendiary incantations."

But the full context of Marley's reference to "bombing a church" in "Talkin' Blues" is repressed. The righteous anger of the oppressed is what motivates the explosion, and the daring to stare into the sun can be read as a sign of supernatural empowerment:

I've been down on the rock so long
I seem to wear a permanent screw
But I'm gonna stare in the sun,
Let the rays shine in my eyes[13]

Further, there is a subtle difference between what Marley actually says, "bombing a church," and the misquote "bombing the church." Any church will do, for what Marley bewails is really a profound sense of the loss of faith in organized religion:

> I'm gonna take a just a one step more
>
> Cause I feel like bombing a church
>
> Now that you know that the preacher is lying
>
> So who's gonna stay at home
>
> When the freedom fighters are fightin?[14]

Despite Marley's perception of the betrayal of the people by the collective church, he can nevertheless take refuge in the comfort of the scriptures. For "Talkin Blues" opens with a biblical allusion—Jacob fleeing from the wrath of his brother Esau, as recorded in Genesis 28:11: "And he [Jacob] lighted upon a certain place, and tarried there all night, because the sun was set; and he took of the stones of that place, and put them for his pillows, and lay down in that place to sleep." The "rock," Jacob's pillow of stones, also alludes to Jamaica itself, which in popular discourse is often referred to as "the rock" or "Jamrock"—thus signifying the hardness of life for many Jamaicans living on the rock and on the edge.

One man's "metaphoric reference" is another's "incendiary incantation." The emotive phrase "incendiary incantations" applied to Sizzla's lyrics connotes both illegal acts of arson and savage, demonic rites. It is no longer a simple matter of a fiery metaphor innocently used by a Bob Marley who, in any case, is really a "One Love" pacifist. The *Oxford English Dictionary (OED)* defines "incendiary" as "1. consisting in, or pertaining to, the malicious setting on fire of buildings or other property. . . . 2. *fig[urative]* Tending to stir up strife, violence or sedition; inflammatory." "Incantation" is defined as "the use of a formula of words spoken or chanted to produce a magical effect; the utterance of a spell or charm; more widely, the use of magical ceremonies or arts; sorcery, enchantment." And sorcery, defined as "the use of magic or enchantment; the practice of magic arts; witchcraft," takes us straight to witchcraft, which the OED defines as: "The practices of a witch or witches; the exercise of supernatural powers supposed to be possessed by persons in league with the devil or evil spirits." So there you have it. Abracadabra! The demonization of Sizzla. Even if one concedes that the *L.A. Times* journalist may have been using "incendiary" in the purely metaphoric sense, "tending to stir up strife, violence or sedition," Sizzla's chant, unlike Bob Marley's, leads directly to literal acts of violence—in and out of church. It cannot orchestrate one love. But what of the less incendiary songs in Sizzla's repertoire, such as "Black Woman and Child"? Why are these excluded in simple-minded evaluations of the DJ's message?

Careful listening to the "One Love" lyrics produces a reading of Bob Marley's message that is much more complicated than first appears. The lyrics of "One Love/People Get Ready," with input from Curtis Mayfield, actually question in part the possibility of "one love." While the I-Three chorus, in parentheses, somewhat optimistically chants "one heart, one love," Bob Marley, the lead singer, seems less certain:

> Let them all pass their dirty remarks (one love)
>
> There is one question I'd really love to ask (one heart)
>
> Is there a place for the hopeless sinner
>
> Who has hurt all mankind just to save his own?
>
> Believe (one love)
>
> What about the "one heart"? (one heart)
>
> What about "let's get together and feel alright"?[15]

What about it? That's the question. Is it possible? How does one accommodate "the hopeless sinner" in the communion of "one love"? That is the challenge. Peace and love require justice. So Marley exhorts: "Let's get together to fight this holy armagideon [*sic*] (one love)/ So when the Man comes there will be no no doom."[16] Marley's "one love" optimism includes a dread reminder of Armageddon, the site of the last decisive battle of the forces of good and evil on the Day of Judgment, referred to in Revelation 16:16.

The Jamaica Tourist Board's decision to adopt and adapt Marley's "One Love" to market the island as a vacation paradise is understandable. It is very difficult to use blood and fire to promote the Jamaican tourist product—unless one is advertising a sizzling jerk meat festival. So it makes commercial sense to construct the fiction of Jamaica as an out-of-many-one paradise. But even a sanitized Rastaman singing "One Love" turned out to be too unlovely a representation of Jamaica for certain backward elements in the society. When the tourist board's "One Love" advertising campaign was first launched in the early 1990s, there was definite resistance in some conservative quarters to the image of a reggae-singing Rastaman as the voice of Jamaica in the overseas market.

In a cynical article entitled "Tourism Madness," columnist Dawn Ritch savaged the "One Love" ad:

> I understand the Jamaica Tourist Board's (JTB's) television commercial was vetted and approved by the Cabinet of Jamaica. Everybody knows that the slogan is "One love, one heart, come to Jamaica and feel awright." I haven't seen the commercial, but reports are that it has flora, fauna and Dunn's River. A more perceptive comment from a veteran hotelier, however, is that the ad seeks to promote Jamaican culture through the use of reggae music, and a Rastafarian musician flashing his locks on stage. The hotelier said, "The Rasta has white teeth, red gums, looks exactly like a gorilla and the Tourist Board would be well-advised not to show it in the Mid-West to white farmers who want what every other Caribbean destination is promoting . . . not culture, but sun, sea and fun. The problem with the Jamaican authorities is that the moment they hear reggae, their hearts begin to beat faster and market sense flies out the window." . . .

Even when reggae was hot, the JTB never used it. Now when the posses have created a perception in the American mind that reggae plus rasta plus drugs means violence, we have a national commercial which reinforces that perception. It may appeal to some corners of the North East, and reggae fans everywhere, but we don't need advertising to bring that market here. They come anyway.[17]

Ritch's secondhand account of the ad is not to be trusted. I have not been able to locate in the Jamaica Tourist Board library any ad that fits the description of a Rasta with "white teeth, red gums, looking exactly like a gorilla." The one Rastafari image in the videos I did see was a long shot of a silhouetted Rastaman, carrying a little child on his back. The child appeared to be white. This may be a revised version of the original close-up shot of the "gorilla." Then again, it may simply be that in the eyes of our unnamed hotelier, any Rastaman, or any Black man for that matter, just naturally looks like a gorilla. Bob Marley's "One Love," appropriated by the Jamaica Tourist Board to project a nonthreatening image of an unequivocally unified Jamaica, is undermined in the eyes of Dawn Ritch's anonymous hotelier-informant by unsettling images of Black bestiality. What an irony!

Professor the Honorable Rex Nettleford, vice-chancellor of the University of the West Indies, gave a characteristically pithy response to Ritch's column, entitled "War, Recession and Gorillas (Tourism Madness Indeed!)" Identifying himself as "one who qualifies for being a gorilla,"[18] he proceeds to disclose the rank racism and stark class prejudice that lurk in Ritch's ill-tempered account of the "One Love" ad:

For the bottom-line we are expected to keep lying to the visitors (from the Mid-West and the South Ms Ritch insists) that there are no black people in Jamaica. And if we admit that there are, they are to be seen merely as smiling waiters, barmen, skulleryboys, chambermaids, beach pimps, entertainers, or muscle-bound life-savers, with a few "Uncle Toms" scattered all over the properties as second-tier managers or some "uppity niggers" stashed away in far-off Kingston where such presumptuous things as daring to govern a country, writing columns for newspapers, or running a University, other education institutions and businesses, are pursued without much success despite the kind efforts of the IMF.[19]

In the early years of the evolution of reggae music—gorilla/guerrilla music—its creators had no need to worry that their distinctive concrete jungle sound, with all its weight of oppression, would be appropriated and misinterpreted by Babylon. It is popularly believed that government institutions such as the Jamaica Tourist Board made it a firm policy *not* to use reggae music to advertise the island. This *raga-raga, buguyaga* music certainly did not conform to the image of Jamaica that was being constructed for tourist consumption. The new nation's motto, "Out of many, one people," served to consolidate an idealized view of Jamaica as a multiracial paradise in which all would feel welcome: one love.

The out-of-many oneness of the tourist board's versions of local social reality, mass-marketed for foreign consumption, is expressed in the unquestioningly positive new lyrics for Bob Marley's far more equivocal song:

Feel Jamaica move you
Warm Jamaica touch you
Hear Jamaica singing
See Jamaica smiling
Feel Jamaica's magic
Hear Jamaica's music
Come to Jamaica and feel alright.[20]

Feel-good reggae as background music *was* all right. But the culture of reggae, encoding the whole history of oppression and exploitation of the masses of the Jamaican people, was not. Apocalyptic reggae lyrics that evoked the imminent collapse of Babylon could not be allowed to penetrate the consciousness of the stereotypical carefree tourist.

But hard-core reggae is above all a politicized music; it challenges abusive manifestations of church and state power. In the words of Marley's

"One Drop," as distinct from "One Love," reggae music is "a rhythm resisting against the system."[21] And reggae is lyrics articulating in both literal and metaphorical language resistance against the brutalizing system. For example, we hear this explosively in "Burnin' and Lootin'," from the 1973 *Burnin'* album. Here the fire is both literal and metaphorical: burning and looting—literal fire; but also burning pollution and illusions—metaphorical fire.

> This morning I woke up in a curfew
> Oh God, I was a prisoner too, yeah
> Could not recognise the faces standing over me
> They were all dressed in uniforms of brutality
> How many rivers do we have to cross
> Before we can talk to the boss?
> All that we got seems lost
> We must have really paid the cost
> That's why we gonna be
> Burnin and a lootin tonight
> One more thing
> Burnin all pollution tonight
> Oh yeah, yeah
> Burnin all illusions tonight.[22]

I too now burn two illusions with one fire: The first illusion is that there is no fire in Bob Marley's metaphor; the second is that there is no metaphor in the DJs' fire. I compare the use of the image of fire in the lyrics of Bob Marley and Capleton and establish the line of affiliation. I choose Capleton, the self-styled Fire Man, as the representative of a whole generation of DJs who create lyrics in Jamaican, a language that is highly charged with metaphor. And I choose the image of fire because it has such universally powerful resonances. In the culture-specific Jamaican context, the fire that burns in the lyrics of both Bob Marley and Capleton is an essential element of Rastafari discourse. As the Mystic Revelation of Rastafari remind us, "Rastaman a fire man." "Peace and Love" and fiery "judgment" have equal place in Rastafari cosmology.

Reggae singer Niney warns in "Blood and Fire" that "Judgement has come and mercy has gone."[23] A somewhat cryptic note to the song in the *Tougher than Tough* Island Records 1993 compilation discloses the way in which allusions to blood and fire in Jamaican popular music are often both literal and metaphorical: "A huge Jamaican hit over Christmas 1970, this militant song ['Blood and Fire'] established Niney as a distinctive voice in reggae. Niney's dub of the tune actually caused a fight between him and organist Glen Adams, who claimed it was lifted from the Wailers' song 'Fire Fire.' When the producer turned up at the pressing plant with the master he was still covered in blood."[24]

The apocalyptic fire of Rastafari—"Lightning earthquake brimstone and fire for the wicked in high and low places!"—clearly has its genesis in the Bible. Alexander Cruden's *Complete Concordance to the Old and New Testament,* first published in London in 1737, identifies approximately 182 references to fire in the Bible and directs readers to the related headings: "brimstone, burn or burnt, coals, consume, consuming, devour, devoured, devouring, flame, hell, midst."[25] More fire. Cruden characterizes this biblical fire thus:

> Is one of the four elements, which not only affords light and heat, but whereby likewise we try and purge metals. God hath often appeared in fire, and encompassed with fire, as when he shewed himself in the burning bush, and descended on mount Sinai in the midst of flames, thunderings, and lightning.
>
> Our Saviour is compared to fire. . . . The Holy Ghost likewise is compared to fire. . . .
>
> Fire from heaven fell frequently on the victims sacrificed to the Lord as a mark of his presence and approbation.
>
> The torments of hell are described by fire, both in the Old and New Testaments.

> The word of God is compared to fire. . . . It is full of life and efficacy; like
> a fire it warms, melts and heals my people, and is powerful to consume the
> dross, and burn up the chaff and stubble. And the apostle says, that every
> man's doctrine should be tried by fire, that is, by the light of the word, of what
> nature it is, whether it be true or false, sound and solid, or corrupt and frothy.
> Fire is likewise taken for persecution, dissension and division.[26]

In Bob Marley's use of the fire image in "Revolution," for example,
issues of social justice rather than religion are primary. The opening lines
of the song may allude to the book of Revelation: "Revelation reveals the
truth, Revelation." But the truth that is revealed is the need for revolution
of a political, not religious nature:

> It takes a revolution
> To make a solution
> Too much confusion
> So much frustration.[27]

This song could very well be taken up as an anthem for the many street
people in Jamaica who are victims of injustice in high and low places:

> I doan wanna live in the park
> Can't trust no shadows after dark
> So, my friend, I wish that you could see
> Like the bird in the tree
> The prisoners must be free, yeah![28]

Politicians who oversee systems of institutionalized oppression are identified as dangerous allies:

> Never make a politician
> Grant you a favour

> They will always want to
> Control you forever[29]

It is these frustrating, confusing conditions that require revolution, and so the *fire-bun* images vividly evoke the destruction of the unjust social order: "So if a fire mek i bun/ And if a blood mek i run."[30] The use of "so" and "if" is intriguing: *If a so, a so* [If that's how it's going to be, well then]. Marley's choice of "if" suggests the possibility that it doesn't have to come to that. If we have a social conscience, we can make the necessary changes in the arrangement of things to ensure positive outcomes. But if we do not, then fire and blood are the inevitable consequences. The insistent "mek i" suggests forces that operate beyond control once they are unleashed. There is also a proverbial quality to the statement that reinforces the sense of inevitability: natural justice running its course.

In "Ride Natty Ride," from the 1979 *Survival* album, fire similarly evokes apocalypse, the implosion of the social order:

> Now the fire is burning
> Out of control, panic in the city
> Wicked weeping for their gold
> Everywhere the fire is burning
> Destroying and melting their gold
> Destroying and wasting their souls.[31]

But, somewhat paradoxically, fire also represents an all-consuming self-knowledge that motivates the Rastaman on his righteous mission and that cannot be destroyed by the forces of oppression. So the fire of destruction is also the source of rekindled creative energy:

> All an all yu see a gwaan
> Is to fight against the Rastaman
> So they build their world in great confusion

To force on us the devil's illusion

But the stone that the builder refuse

Shall be the head cornerstone

And no matter what games they play

There is something they can never take away

And it's the fire, it's the fire

Fire burning down everything

Feel the fire, fire, the fire, the fire

Only the birds have wings

No time to be deceived

You should know and not believe

Jah says this judgement could never be with water

So no water could put out this fire

This fire, this fire

Go deh dready, go deh, dready, go deh![32]

Careful listeners can readily hear echoes of Bob Marley's explosive fire in Capleton's lyrics. But because the pace of delivery of the DJ's lyrics is of Courtney Walshian velocity, at times it is difficult for the inattentive ear to perceive the continuities between Capleton's and Bob Marley's chant against Babylon.[33] Liner notes with transcriptions of the oral text facilitate full comprehension, but these transcriptions must be accurate. It is amusing to read some of the mistranscriptions of even Marley's lyrics. For example, in "Get Up, Stand Up," from the Wailers' *Burnin'* album, the line "We're sick and tired of your ism schism game," sung by Tosh, who coauthored the song, becomes in transcription the nonsensical "We're sick and tired of your easing kissing game." And this is supposedly the authorized version of the written text. In "Revolution," the line "Kill cramp an paralyze all weak-heart conception" becomes the politically incorrect "Kill cramp and paralyze all weak at conception."

The liner notes to Capleton's *More Fire* CD on the VP Records label do not include transcriptions of the oral text. Nevertheless, the notes are useful because they locate Capleton's fire within a wider biblical and African-diasporic discourse of burning references. Eight quotations are given from: the book of Daniel in the Bible; H Rap Brown; abolitionist William Lloyd Garrison; Peter Tosh; Bob Marley (twice); Rasta (generic); and the Wailers. A cultural, political, and ideological frame for Capleton's use of fire on this CD is thus defined. Herbie Miller, who produced the CD, is responsible for selecting the quotations. But one should not make the mistake of assuming that Capleton could not have done so himself. Some DJs are very well read and do understand the wide political influences that shape their own lyrical performances.

Just one example will suffice. Early one Sunday morning, Buju Banton came to my home looking for a copy of John Jackson's *Introduction to African Civilization*. He wanted to borrow the book for some youths who were participating in an innovative reading group promoted by the inventive Andrea Williams-Green, presenter of the extremely popular "Running African" program on IRIE FM. Buju also borrowed for himself Cheik Anta Diop's *The African Origins of Civilization*. The many folk philosophers in Jamaican society who read widely and purely for knowledge and pleasure—not just to get a piece of paper that will presumably qualify them for jobs—put to shame many university students, who merely want to get through as little of the required reading for their courses as possible.

The quotations on Capleton's *More Fire* are from:

1. The book of Daniel: "Shadrack, Meshach and Abednego walked through fire and never got burned."
2. H. Rap Brown: "Burn, baby, burn."
3. William Lloyd Garrison: "I have need to be all on fire for I have mountains of ice about me to melt."
4. Peter Tosh: "Fire, fire, Babylon burning"
5. Bob Marley: "Slave Driver, the tables have turned/ Catch a fire, you're gonna get burned."
6. Bob Marley: "So if a fire mek it bun an if a blood mek it run"[34]

7. Rasta: "Lightning, earthquake, brimstone and fire for all the wicked in high and low places!"

8. The Wailers: "Burnin an a-lootin tonight. Burning all illusion tonight."

And beneath all of those quotes, in the boldest of all the fonts, is "Word Sound Power."

The first of the twenty chants on the *More Fire* CD, appropriately entitled "Fire Chant," is a wonderfully witty mix of both literal and metaphorical allusions to fire. It begins with a surprising inversion—a bottom's-up, setting on its head of the Jamaican bad word *raas claat:* "Holy Emmanuel I, Selassie I. Talk to raas, youth! Mi seh fi talk to raas! Talk to Raas Tafari! Unu hear weh mi seh? Mi seh unu fi talk to raas claat! Hold on! Through unu hear mi seh 'raas claat' unu tink is indecent language. Always remember seh di word 'Ras' mean 'head' and check mi turban an mi claat dat tie it. Seet? So mi seh 'raas cleat.'"[35]

The tail—*raas*—becomes the head—Ras—and the DJ thus claims for Rastafari the dread power to simultaneously neutralize and reenergize so-called bad words. What is particularly amusing in Capleton's "cloth of the Ras" word-play is the way in which the DJ seems quite content to metaphorically put on his head the *raas claat* (menstrual cloth) that literally is placed on a woman's private parts. Capleton's gendered inversion thus suggests a quite revolutionary Rastafari body politics: subverting the female "low" and making it "high." I sincerely hope Capleton will not *fire bun* me for this mischievous rereading of his own act of subversion.

The "Fire Chant" proceeds in a less provocative mode to explicate how Capleton uses the metaphor of fire in his work. He illustrates with great humor the many uses of fire and concludes by drawing a connection between the fiery rhetoric of Christian hymns and sermons and his own rhetorical fire:

Jamaican:

Well di fire is fi di purification an how di fo . . . how can you fight against fire? When yu wake up inna di morning an yu want a cup of tea, is fire, don't? Inna di evening, yu waan some food. A still fire.

So mi seh mi bun car an some man a talk bout "how yu fi bun car an yu drive car?" Den yu no understand weh mi mean or yu no overstand? Mi seh mi bun car mean seh yu mustn't put car in front of humanity. Dat mean yu must see yu brothers an sister before yu see car. Becau people is more valuable than material.

But if yu a gwaan like yu waan complicated or been ridiculous with yu lickle mental capacity, mi no a go mek yu know! Yu waan mi get evil wid di fire? Well, anytime I go into my car, fron [sic] I drive car I have to bun it. Cau remember when mi press gas, a bun mi a bun gas. Yu know dat. And when mi press mi brake, a bun mi a bun brake also. When mi turn on mi ignition, yu know how much fire dat inna mi engine? If I need some music an turn on mi stereo, a fire gi mi dat. But, watch di bigger judgement! If ah need some cool aircondition, a fire generate dat also. So always remember seh di fire is the main source of life.

Mi pass di church an mi hear dem deh pon "Keep di fire burnin." Hear dem again, "A lickle more oil in my lamp, keep it burnin." Hear dem noh, "God nah come back wid no water; a brimstone an fire." Den wa di fo unu confuse bout fire? Fire is for di purification.

Unu waan know sopn? Di herb heal. But is still di fire ha fi burn di herb so di herb coulda able fi heal. Watch ya again! Di water cleanse. But a still di fire ha fi burn di water an purify di water so di water coulda able fi cleanse. Any man weh no have no fire, dead! Holy Emmanuel I, Selassie I.[36]

English:
Well the fire is for the purification and how the fo . . . how can you fight against fire? When you wake up in the morning and want a cup of tea, it's fire, isn't it? In the evening, you want some food. It's still fire.

So I say that I burn car; and some people are asking "how can you burn car and you drive a car?" Don't you understand what I mean or don't you overstand? When I say that I burn car that means you mustn't put car in front of humanity. That means you must see your brothers and sisters before you see car. Because people are more valuable than material objects.

But if you want to complicate matters, or if you're being ridiculous and don't have the mental capacity to understand what I'm saying, let me explain! Do you want me to demonstrate how bad I am in my use of fire? Well, whenever I go in my car to drive, I have to burn it. Because, just remember, when I press the gas pedal, I'm burning gas. You do know that. And when I press my brake, I'm also burning brakes. When I turn on my ignition, do you know how much fire there is in my engine? If I need some music and turn on my stereo, it's fire again that gives it to me. But consider this paradox! If I need some cool air conditioning, it's fire that generates it also. So always remember that fire is the main source of life.

I pass a church and I hear them repeatedly saying "Keep the fire burning." Listen to them again: "A little more oil in my lamp, keep it burning." Hear them: "God is not coming back with water; it's brimstone and fire." Then why the fo are you confused about fire? Fire is for purification.

Do you want to know something? The herb heals. But it is still the fire that has to burn the herb so that the herb is able to heal. Listen to this! The water cleanses. But it is still the fire that has to burn the water and purify the water so that the water is able to cleanse. Any man who doesn't have fire is dead! Holy Emmanuel I, Selassie I.

In another chant, "I Am," the "Intro" to Capleton's 1999 *One Mission* CD, one can hear echoes of Bob Marley's "Ambush in the Night," which says:

They say what we know is just what they teach us
And we're so ignorant cause every time they can reach us
Through political strategy they keep us hungry
And when you gonna get some food
Your brother got to be your enemy

...

Well, what we know is not what they tell us

We're not ignorant, I mean it

And they just cannot touch us

Through the powers of the most high

We keep on surfacing

Through the powers of the most high

We keep on surviving.[37]

Capleton affirms the very same conviction:

Capleton is all about, you know, righteousness and, you know, upliftment a di nation an di people. Becau yu done know, Babylon try limit I and I as a nation a people, you know weh me a seh [what I'm saying]. Even pon a educational levels. Weh dem give yu "O" levels and PhDs an den dem lock you off inna a corner and seh "yeow, whatever I taught you, you know, dat's what you know." But the real authentic thing weh yu fi know bout yuself [that you should know about yourself] as a race an a nation a people in terms of heritage and culture and philosophies and curriculum, that [is] never taught inna di school nor di institution nor di college, you know. So you intend to [so it is intended that you] become limited. Yu know weh I mean? But I & I see I self pon an unlimited level. You know weh I mean? I & I look pon life from a nature-al aspect of life. So everything weh I & I see in front a [of] I & I it have to be real. So I couldn't get caught up inna the disillusion an di fantasy.[38]

Similarly, in "More Prophet," Capleton, like Marley, burns both illusion and disillusion:

People dem a bawl seh dem [that they] want more prophet

Di corruption an di slackness

A di prophet come fi [to]stop it

Dem a bawl seh dem want more prophet

Disillusion an confusion a di prophet come fi bun it

. . .

Fire ha fi usè [must be used] fi bun out confusion

Bun dis-illusion an bun temptation

Mek dem know di fire is fi di purification.[39]

I hyphenate "dis-illusion" because it is not entirely clear if Capleton intends us to hear "dis illusion" or "disillusion"—or a compound of both meanings. The context allows both the Jamaican Creole "dis illusion" [this illusion] and the English "disillusion."

The most problematic of Capleton's fiery chants that I examine here is "Hunt You." I confess that I feel decided discomfort with the predatory intensity of the DJ's hunt for the objects of his desire. This is decidedly not a case of waiting in vain:

I'm hunting to find, I'm hunting to find,

I'm hunting to find

A natural girl that is mine, yeah

Black uman [woman] mi a hunt yu, hunt yu, hunt yu

Any day now mi ready fi upfront yu.[40]

Admittedly, in matters of sexual politics, it is often difficult to distinguish between hunter and prey. Women have been socialized to hunt men while seeming to be mere prey. And, in any case, most women do not mind being vigorously hunted by a man they desire. It is the hunt of the undesired predator that is frightening.

Like Shabba Ranks with his trailer load of girls, Capleton is hunting girls in packs of ten and twenty:

Jamaican:

Right ya now mi seh mi waan di uman dem plenty

Gi mi dem inna tens an inna twenty

Uman alone mi seh mi want inna mi documentary
Inna mi country a uman alone a get entry
Hunt dem from London straight to Coventry
From St Mary straight to Senti
No time at all mi bedroom no fi empty[41]

English:
Right now I want women in abundance
Give them to me in bunches of tens and twenty
I'm saying that I want only women in my documentary
In my country only women are allowed entry
Hunt them from London straight to Coventry
From St. Mary straight to Senti
At no time at all must my bedroom be empty

Somewhat surprisingly, the DJ does pause in the heat of the hunt to celebrate the woman's right to be treated with respect by men. Indeed, the "you" addressed in the following lines seems to be all of the women hunted and, simultaneously, the DJ's "special" woman who deserves particular care:

Fire fi a bwoy if a dump im waan dump yu
[Fire for the boy who wants to dump you]
. . .
After yu [you are] no hog fi no bwoy come grunt yu
After yu no tyre fi no bwoy come pump yu
After yu no punk fi no bwoy come punk yu
After yu no circus fi no bwoy come stunt yu
After yu no cart fi no bwoy come chump yu
After yu no garbage fi no bwoy come dump yu
After yu no fence fi no bwoy come jump yu
Hey, see di Prophet chariot deh fi upfront yu![42]

[Hey, see the Prophet's chariot there to elevate you!]

In addition, the DJ's heterosexist zeal makes him *fire bun* homosexuals—male and female; and his puritanical streak makes him *fire bun,* as well, sexual practices of which he disapproves: oral and anal sex. It is all quite explicit:

Jamaican:

Only funny man alone woulda waan bump yu

Fire fi a bwoy if im waan fi backbench yu

. . .

Uman no waan no man fi eat off her . . .

Seh she want a man fi mek her rail an jump

Seh she want a man fi gi her di tree trunk

Fire fi di bwoy weh go eat it like lunch

Fire fi di bwoy weh drink it like fruit punch

Fire should go put pon di booger man stunt

Fire should go put pon dem lesbian stunt

Diss black uman an know di judgment a bos.[43]

English:

Only a queer would want to bump you

Fire upon a boy if he wants to backbench you

. . .

Women don't want men to eat off her . . .

I say, she wants a man to make her gyrate

I say, she wants a man to give her the tree trunk

Fire upon the boy who goes and eats it like lunch

Fire upon the boy who drinks it like fruit punch

Fire should be put on the queer man's stunt

Fire should be put on those lesbians' stunt

If you disrespect Black women, know that judgment will fall.

This is one of the areas in which some of the younger-generation of DJs could learn from Bob Marley. Whereas Marley often used proverbial wisdom to chant down Babylon—throwing word without naming names; throwing corn without calling fowl—the youths not only throw corn, *dem call fowl, dem catch the fowl, dem wring off di fowl neck, dem pick the feathers and dump the carcass in a pot of boiling water on the fire.* But even Marley was tempted to be explicit in his name-calling. While he may deny calling fowl, "throw mi corn, mi no call no fowl,"[44] he immediately undercuts that assertion by voicing the traditional fowl call "mi saying coop, coop, coop, cluck, cluck, cluck."[45]

It is clear from this comparative analysis of the use of fire imagery in the lyrics of Bob Marley and Capleton that there are continuities between the work of both men as well as differences. The anger and the frustration with Babylon system are almost identical. What is different is the *riddim* of the rage. If we listen carefully we can hear. Capleton reminds us that our educational institutions ought to teach "the real authentic thing weh wi ha fi know bout wiself as a race, as a nation an a people in terms of heritage an culture an philosophies an curriculum." And Bob Marley similarly warned:

> Babylon system is the vampire
> Sucking the children day by day
> Babylon system is the vampire
> Sucking the blood of the sufferers
> Building church and university
> Deceiving the people continually.[46]

Bob Marley exhorts us to "tell di children di truth."[47] Each generation must tell its own complex truth. And, truth be told, if Marley were a youth today, he would sound a lot like Capleton: "More Fire."

"Vile Vocals"

Exporting Jamaican
Dancehall Lyrics to Barbados

Dancehall has been much more notorious than any other Caribbean popular music form in terms of its perceived support for activities that can give rise to the AIDS epidemic.[1]

—Curwen Best

Dub and Ragga music also offers [*sic*] a pathway into the inscape of terminality. Simultaneously ultramodern, fin de siècle and primitive, Dub and Ragga, like their cousin African-American Rap, are "songs of the skeleton."[2]

—Gordon Rohlehr

These epigraphs, arising from the work of two scholars of Caribbean popular music—Best from Barbados and Rohlehr from Guyana (now long resident in Trinidad)—exemplify the bad press that Jamaican dancehall music often suffers in the eastern Caribbean. Reduced to skeletal emaciation, the stricken body of song texts cannot stand up to prolonged scrutiny. From within the academy as well as without comes a babble of censorious voices conspiring to deny the art form its full range of contradictory meaning, indiscriminately chanting down and dubbing over the lyrics of the DJs. Focusing on Caribbean regional issues, this chapter examines some of the ideological implications of the widespread disvaluation of Jamaican popular music (emphasis on the *diss*) and contrasts the divisive nationalist discourses of the region's elites with the populist, pan-Caribbean identity that is affirmed in popular music circulating freely beyond national borders.

The hue and cry raised in the Barbadian media in response to an April 2000 Caribbean Broadcasting Union (CBU) *Talk Caribbean* television program on Jamaican dancehall/dub lyrics is an excellent example of the hysteria that frank discussion of popular culture often provokes. Especially when the cultural product is exported and, in the process, stripped of its layers of indigenous meaning, it becomes subject to much misinterpretation in its new context of appropriation. The public outcry in Barbados against dancehall music and its articulate apologists noisily demands censorship of the "muck, the raw incitement to rebellion and violence which loom large on the 'dub' menu." Mixed metaphor aside, this quote from the *Barbados Advocate* editorial of April 11, 2000, denotes the purist construction of national identity in elitist Barbadian discourses. "Barbados" is conceived immaculately; "Jamaica" is synonymous with sin.

The contemptuous headline of the editorial, "Vile Vocals," and its combative subtitle, "Unofficial War in Bim," are an aggressive declaration of intent to defend Barbadian hegemony against the encroachments of Jamaican culture in its many treacherous forms. Indeed, "Vile Vocals" refers not only to the "impure" content of the lyrics but also to the moral depravity of the "bastardized" Jamaican Creole language in which the villainous vocals are voiced. Any attempt to encourage Barbadians to learn Jamaican so that they can be sure of the meaning of lyrics they are condemning is itself misconstrued as an immoral act.

This impassioned editorial exemplifies the irrationality that undermines much of the public discourse on Jamaican "dub" music in Barbados today. Beginning with an attack on the Creole language in the United States—a language that is indeed related to Jamaican Creole—the planto-cratic editorial asserts that acknowledging the intrinsic worth of Creole languages as useful is an acceptance of the "supposed intellectual inferiority" of their habitual speakers. In Jamaica one hears this reductionist argument all the time. One of its most disdainful exponents was Morris Cargill, the senior columnist of Jamaica's centuries-old newspaper, the *Gleaner,* who died in 2000. Cargill was notorious for his attacks on Jamaican Creole, which he scornfully termed "yahoolish." Listen to his dog, who ostensibly wrote a column for him that was published on February 25, 1999: "one of the aims of my society is to develop a proper understanding of dog language. If people can propose that what my man calls yahoolish should become a second language in Jamaica I see no reason why poodlese should not become a third one. It is, after all, at least as understandable."

The *Talk Caribbean* program clearly illustrates a Barbadian failure to understand the preferred language of Jamaican dancehall lyrics. One of the panelists on the program, David Ellis, an upstanding broadcaster at the Starcom Network News radio station in Barbados, defines dancehall lyrics as essentially unintelligible, especially to older ears. The base beat becomes the sole signifier: "It is a music with a reggae base whose lyrical content is very difficult to understand. I think many people sum it up that way. And that's the challenge that many people in the Caribbean have with it. Older people just do not understand the lyrics. And it is in that environment that some younger people exploit the ignorance."[3]

I agree with Ellis that age is a key variable in determining the intelligibility of dancehall lyrics—in Jamaica as much as elsewhere in the Caribbean. Dancehall is, essentially, a youth music. And the youths who chant verbatim in tune with the performances of their favorite superstars celebrate communal rituals of mutual understanding. But other factors must be taken into account in explaining why dancehall's "lyrical content" is so difficult for some listeners, many of whom would even deny that there is any "content" in the lyrics. An immediate obscurity arises from the audience's incompetence in the Jamaican Creole language. Then there are the limitations of (un)intelligibility that class arrogance imposes. And there are the prejudices that intolerant religious passion aggravates.

Despite Ellis's disclaimer, he nevertheless proceeds from a position of near-total adult ignorance to vilify lyrics that he obviously does not understand. For example, condemning Mr. Vegas's "She's a Ho" because of its vulgar use of the earthy, African-Americanized Anglo-Saxon word "whore," Ellis fails to hear the DJ's strident critique of prostitution. Incidentally, like many a whore, the word "whore" itself has gone down in life. The *Oxford English Dictionary* (*OED*) gives its etymology as the Latin "carus," meaning "dear." And it is true that many dearly beloved whores, especially at the top end of the market, are very dear indeed. The dictionary notes that "whore is now confined to coarse and abusive speech, exc[ept] in occasional echoes of historical expression, as the whore of Babylon." Polite society prefers the latinate "prostitute," "Pro + statuere to cause to stand." In these feminist times, even prostitute is no longer politically correct; the preferred term is the gender-neutral "sex worker," an occupation that is no less precarious for the euphemism.

Problems of intelligibility immediately arise in the *Talk Caribbean* program with the inaccurate transcription of lyrics that distorts Mr. Vegas's meaning. Viewers who cannot decode the lyrics in the fluid moment of performance become dependent on the "fixed" visual text that, in this instance, reproduces misunderstanding.

For example, in the transcription of the line in "She's a Ho" that denounces loose women who have sex in quick succession with two men in the same night, the "two" is omitted, thus making nonsense of the DJ's principled stand against promiscuity, not sex. Again, the DJ's rebuke of the woman who, in a remarkable analogy, is uncharitably compared to a clothespin—needing very little persuasion to open her legs to all and sundry—is not transcribed accurately. What Mr. Vegas actually says is that one of the woman's many partners dies and no one knows what kills him—an allusion to AIDS, the seemingly unspeakable terminal illness. The erroneous transcription omits the "not," converting the not knowing into its very opposite. It thus completely effaces the DJ's meaning. A relatively minor matter is the error in transcription of the man's name that is represented as "Bum," not "Bim." But the inaccuracy confirms the transcriber's consistent inattention to detail.

The following couplet, which deepens the meaning of the weight loss reference, is thoroughly garbled: "Sleep wid Bim, Bim dead/ An dem don't know a wha kill im" [She slept with Bim, Bim is dead/ And nobody knows what caused his death]. The not knowing, which is clearly intended as an allusion to unmentionable AIDS, is entirely lost in the mistranscription which becomes "Sleep wid Bum, him dead/ An dem know a what kill him." [She slept with Bum; he's dead/ And they know what caused his death.] In the ensuing exchange between myself and Ellis during the program a number of provocative issues arose. My attempt, as interpreter, to locate Mr. Vegas's lyrics within an intelligible biblical discourse—a sacrosanct context that would legitimize the use of the word whore as an "occasional echo of an historical expression, such as the whore of Babylon"—to evoke the lexical, if not moral, authority of the OED—was dismissed. Ellis, the voice of received wisdom and censorship, had already made up his mind. Any reference by Mr. Vegas to "whore" could only signify complete depravity.

The other panelist on the program, Anthony "Admiral" Nelson, made a valiant attempt to function as referee. Throughout the program he called for translation as an obvious strategy to ensure comprehension. Indeed, his definition of dancehall/dub acknowledges both word and beat: "It has some pulsating rhythms, some crude lyrics sometimes, some vulgar lyrics sometimes and I believe that basically it has been very much misinterpreted." Whereas Ellis retreats into self-satisfied ignorance, the much-younger Admiral descries misinterpretation as a regrettable feature of the Barbadian response to Jamaican dancehall lyrics.

The input of the callers to the television program was similarly instructive. From Barbados itself, from St. Vincent, Grenada, and St.

Lucia, both male and female participants contributed their insights to the debate. On the use of the word "whore," one male caller from Barbados noted that some men abusively apply the label to any woman who refuses to respond to unsolicited male advances. The word thus becomes a telling expression of the perverse politics of male disempowerment. Another male caller, this time from St. Vincent, agreed that "She's a Ho" is a "bad song" and elaborated his view of the new culture of the dancehall as an aggressive discourse: "Is no more a dance nor enjoyment; is a total war between the people and the music." Yet another border clash.

Again and again the issue of the unintelligibility of the lyrics arose. An introspective female caller from St. Lucia pondered the meaning of the dissonance of word and beat in dancehall music: "I'm speaking as a twenty-eight-year-old young lady who does go out. Ahm, what happens normally is that we don't understand, well . . . as a young lady I don't understand the . . . the words of a lot of the songs that are normally played. I don't understand them at all. But I know when I do go out—and I go out to dance—it gives me a positive . . . I feel . . . I have more self-confidence I should say, and I don't know why exactly. I just wanted to know why would that happen—I don't know—if it's something so negative." On reading my transcript of the television program, I became intrigued by this caller's insistence that, "as a young lady," she doesn't understand the words of the dancehall songs. I regret having not thought to press her on the matter. I couldn't help wondering if, perhaps, this young woman very well *does* understand some of the Jamaican dancehall lyrics but because her construction of "young ladyness" precludes intimacy with certain forms of verbal vulgarity, she feels constrained to simulate innocence—a familiar female strategy for negotiating the disturbing complexities of sexual knowledge.

I recall Jamaica Kincaid's critique of this "young lady business" in the novel *Annie John*, set in Antigua. There Kincaid evokes the ritual celebration of the body and the illicit pleasures of unladylike calypso songs—akin to Jamaican dancehall lyrics—in which adolescent girls freely participate, unrepressed by the strictures of respectability:

> Each Friday afternoon, the girls in the lower forms were given, instead of a last lesson period, an extra-long recess. We were to use this in lady-like recreation—walks, chats about the novels and poems we were reading, showing each other the new embroidery stitches we had learned to master in home class, or something just as seemly. Instead, some of the girls would play a game of cricket or rounders or stones, but most of us would go to the far end of the school grounds and play band. In this game, of which teachers and parents disapproved and which was sometimes absolutely forbidden, we would place our arms around each other's waist or shoulders, forming lines of ten or so girls, and then we would dance from one end of the school grounds to the other. As we danced, we would sometimes chant these words: "Tee la la la, come go. Tee la la la, come go." At other times we would sing a popular calypso song which usually had lots of unladylike words to it.[4]

Anticipating the St. Lucian young lady's ambivalent testimony, Gordon Rohlehr provides an answer to her plaintive question in the essay "Folk Research: Fossil or Living Bone?" from which the pessimistic, skeletal epigraph to this chapter is taken. Qualifying the rhetoric of terminality, Rohlehr discovers the untainted joy that popular music as communal dance ritual offers its celebrants. Kincaid's carefree girl children in the schoolyard and the much more burdened female caller to the *Talk Caribbean* television program share a long history of resistance to the debilitating strictures of eurocentrism:

> Yet, paradoxically, Dub and Ragga exist and are popular not primarily for their violence, which is taken for granted as a normal feature of an age when anything from CIA-subversion, a stray bullet, a Friday-afternoon coup or AIDS might claim one's life at any time. They are popular because of their celebratory nature, their capacity to generate joy, catharsis and release in the

midst of constant stress. In other words, they fulfil [*sic*] precisely the same function that weekend Dance Assemblies, the oldest social gathering, of the post-Columbian Caribbean, performed for Africans enslaved to the grinding routines of plantation society. There can be no doubt that it is a kind of joy youth seek and find in their massive huddlings together in congregations of 20,000 and 30,000.[5]

Nevertheless, ephemeral, youthful joy evaporates. The paragraph's ending returns us to the melancholy rhetoric of terminality. The amassed congregation, on the brink of extinction, DJs its death knell—a global angst:

This massiveness—and "massive" is one of their words—represents a huddling of the lonely crowd world-wide, a recreation of a kind of collective folk consciousness, as in the Woodstocks and sit-ins of the late sixties and early seventies, but in the mangled context of the post-industrial universe of the detritus of everything that has outlived its original usefulness.[6]

It is this same sense of terminality that pervades the *Barbados Advocate*'s vitriolic "Vile Vocals" editorial, which draws a melodramatic parallel between the fall of ancient world empires and the predicted decline of new-world Bajan civilization if the Jamaicanization process, engendered by the indiscriminate importation of dancehall music, is allowed to run its destructive course. The bombastic editorial grandiloquently denounces dancehall music as "the Trojan Horse of a counter-culture" that will breach the social security of the Barbadian nation state:

. . . perverse indulgence, laxity and complacency ensured decline of powers as diverse as Babylonia and the Roman Empire.

Given some of the nonsense that passes for intellectual insight into the impact of corrosive 'dub' music, one wonders whether Barbados and other

Caribbean societies are not laying themselves open, if not for similar collapse at least for degradation of a sort spawned in Jamaica's ghettoes.[7]

Indeed, it is the spectre of ghettoization/Jamaicanization of Barbadian society that inspires the erection of protective barriers.

There is an uncanny similarity between the current Barbadian demonization of Jamaican dancehall music and the much-earlier Barbadian rejection of jazz in the 1950s. Kamau (formerly Edward) Brathwaite—Barbadian poet, historian, and cultural critic par excellence—relates an amusing anecdote that illustrates the Barbadian elite's perennial contempt for "foreign" musical expressions that taint the cultural purity of the nation. In an interview with Nathaniel Mackey, Brathwaite recalls the public outrage at his participation, as a schoolboy, in a radio broadcast of jazz music:

It was regarded as devil music in Barbados, especially bebop, which I grew up on in the fifties there. We had a radio program as schoolboys—Harrison College, you know, the elite school of the island—and when we went on the air that first evening, the one and only evening, the people flooded the station with phone calls demanding the incarceration of the perpetrators, the, as they saw us, *cultural traitors*. . . . And you can imagine me upon the carpets of the various drawing rooms around the island afterwards: how I had let the "side" upside down (a partial cricket metaphor—Barbados is the HQ of Cricket) and "Harrson" College (Harrson/Harrison College is the HQ of Caribbean Education) and "Cdear Eddie Mahn, you int got no *Shame*," etc, etc, etc, as if I was some slave rebel like Bussa.[8]

Brathwaite's evocation of the Bussa-led revolt against slavery is not a melodramatic overstatement of the revolutionary potential of African diasporic musics to disturb the peace. Cultural noise destabilizes the uneasy balance of power between those who are easily shamed by cultural traitors and those who have no shame. The embarrassed drawing-room condemnation of the jazz program, like the *Advocate* editorial, similarly questions the viability of the premier educational institutions of the region as agencies for effectively reproducing "cultured" graduates who will not shame their country—or, put quite differently, for ensuring the perpetual mental slavery of brainwashed students who are taught to be ashamed of their own cultural traditions.

Given my own location within the academy, I find most disturbing the editorial's interrogation of the permissive politics of the University of the West Indies as a regional institution that valorizes Creole linguistics and popular culture as subjects of intellectual inquiry. In a direct attack on the scholarship that Caribbean linguists and cultural studies academics have been doing at the university for the last several decades, the editorial declaims:

> Like those who favour ebonics for US blacks, she [Cooper] seeks to elevate "dub" by referring to research at the University of the West Indies. Further, she invites Barbadians to learn the vocabulary of "dub" so as to embrace what the vocalists are "singing."
>
> We concede that it is in the nature of University life to be probing, exploratory, of broad mind and vision. Still, universities should be sensitive to the needs and expectations of citizens whose highest purpose they profess to serve. In the past we have raised questions as to how the UWI sees its function in these Caribbean societies, countries delicately poised between progress and peril to an extent much greater than obtains in powerful, resilient USA.[9]

"[S]ensitive to the needs and expectations" of the many constituencies that the regional institution serves, Professor the Honorable Rex Nettleford, vice-chancellor of the University of the West Indies, nevertheless does acknowledge the centrality of the university's role in the urgent enterprise of cultural decolonization in our small-island states. Thus, he defines the study of Caribbean popular culture as a process of "rethinking the classics."[10] This rethinking, as Nettleford elaborates, requires a revaluation of the privileged cultural hierarchy of aesthetic values in the contemporary Caribbean. Conventional wisdom constructs a pyramid of aesthetic forms and practices at the top of which is the "classical." The center is occupied by the "contemporary/popular." At the very base is the "folk." Given the racialized history of the Caribbean, it is not surprising that the pyramid is color-coded. The "classical" peak is eurocentric/white; the "folk" base is Afrocentric/Black; the "contemporary/popular" center is a gray area. Although one could very well argue that the base as foundation is the most important structural element of this pyramid, one must nevertheless concede the historical and contemporary devaluation of the base folk in the Caribbean.

Despite the protestations of the *Advocate* ideologues, revaluation of this "debased" culture of the folk and its contemporary manifestations as "popular culture" is an entirely legitimate preoccupation of researchers at the university. Indeed, the emergence of the ambitiously named International Reggae Studies Centre on the Mona campus of the University of the West Indies in Jamaica is an important academic development, which I initiated. The project has its genesis in a long tradition of regional scholarship that focuses on populist consciousness in all its multifariousness. It finds its emotive ideological justification in the exhortatory lyrics of Bob Marley's moving "Redemption Song": "Emancipate yourselves from mental slavery/ None but ourselves can free our minds."[11] Marley, amplifying in song the visionary words of Marcus Garvey, broadens the reach of the philosopher's message. Indeed, this representation of the emancipation process as a freeing of the mind from the tenacious shackles of mental slavery is an artful, streetwise restatement of a familiar academic concept: the redemptive politics of decolonization.

The resonances of "redemption" are potent, as the *OED* definitions make clear: There are the pacifist echoes of Christian redemption— "deliverance from sin and its consequences by the atonement of Jesus Christ." There are, as well, the militant reverberations of Caribbean slave history: redemption as "the action of freeing a prisoner, captive, or slave by payment; ransom." Somewhat ironically, "redemption" in this latter sense—buying out of the dehumanizing slave system—often means liberation from the weight of conservative Christian traditions that valorize the passive acceptance of one's lot in life, with the promise of deferred gratification in the life to come.

Bob Marley expresses in song a tradition of visionary insight, a body of *overstanding* (to use a subversive Rastafari word), that is not always acknowledged as knowledge by the academy. Thus, one of the primary projects of the International Reggae Studies Centre is to bring into the academy the knowledge that is expressed in reggae music as a distinctly Jamaican cultural formation. This process of revaluing native knowledge is intended to highlight the ideological underpinnings of the music itself and facilitate analysis of the relationship between book knowledge and the wisdom of the streets. An equally important project of the center is foregrounded by the modifier "international." The center focuses on the evolution of international reggae—both the "pure" and "hybridized" forms that have emerged from the cross-fertilization of Jamaican reggae with other world musics such as soca.

Further, reggae studies is a multidisciplinary enterprise; it requires the collaboration of a wide range of academics within the university and a diverse group of practitioners in the field to close the perceived gap between the university's purely "academic" preoccupations and the rather practical concerns of the reggae music industry. The challenge the university must confront in fulfilling the mandate of emancipation from mental slavery is pointedly stated by Marley:

> Babylon system is the vampire
> Sucking the blood of the sufferers.
> Building church and university
> Deceiving the people continually.[12]

This representation of the university in the popular imagination as an agent of the vampirish state is one of the barriers that must be negotiated.

Indeed, there is a long-established Rastafari inversion of the original name of the University of the West Indies—University College of the West Indies—abbreviated as UC.[13] In dread talk, "you see," the homonym of UC, becomes "you blind." The vision that is so grandiloquently pronounced in the university's motto, "Lux oriens ex occidente"—"A light rising from the West"—is thus eclipsed in cynical, populist discourse.

"War on Ignorance," my sardonic response to that malevolent *Advocate* editorial, engendered even more acrimony.[14] There I cite George Lamming's 1953 novel, *In the Castle of My Skin,* described by the *New Statesman* as "the fundamental book of a civilisation. . . . Mr. Lamming captures the myth-making and myth-dissolving mind of childhood."[15] That iconoclastic novel anticipates the shamelessly egalitarian, "myth-dissolving" transformation of Barbadian society—independent of any influence of vile dancehall lyrics imported from Jamaica—that is now so passionately lamented by the Barbadian elite. Lamming's Trumper, a migrant laborer newly returned home from the United States, prefigures the many Caribbean youths who find in the musics of the African diaspora a language to express their sense of alienation from societies that have failed to fulfill the promise of, first, emancipation and, then, independence.

G Trumper's distanced childhood companion, does not understand the full meaning of the "my people" whom his enterprising friend has learned to claim in the United States. When Trumper plays on his tape recorder Paul Robeson's rendition of "Let My People Go," he initiates a conversation with G about identity that is now defined in cosmopolitan, racial terms—not in village-bound and purely nationalist frames. G's provincial discomfort is evident in the temptation to deride what he does not comprehend:

"Who are your people?" I asked him. It seemed a kind of huge joke.

"The Negro race." said Trumper. The smile had left his face, and his manner had turned grave again. I finished my drink and looked at him. He

knew that I was puzzled. The bewilderment about Trumper's people was real.
At first I thought he meant the village. This allegiance was something bigger.
I wanted to understand it. He drained the glass and set it on the table.

"I didn't know it till I reach the States," he said.

"Didn't know what?" I insisted. I understood the Negro race perfectly,
but I didn't follow how I was involved. He hadn't spoken.

"Know what?" I insisted. "What did you know there?"

"My people," he said, "or better, my race. 'Twus in the States I find it,
an' I'm gonner keep it till thy kingdom come."[16]

In the light of this exchange, the *Advocate*'s gratuitous reference to
the United States proves decidedly ironic. For the United States, far from
constituting a more balanced, less perilous ideological space than the
Caribbean, is the very locale in which cultural identity, sharply represented in black and white, becomes a site of contestation for certain
marginalized migrants. Trumper's newly discovered Negro spirituals
and the seductive technology of the tape recorder are metaphors for the
amplification of all the musics in the African diaspora—including dub/
dancehall—that give Black people the power to say "let my people go."
Admittedly, the tempo and lyrics of Jamaican dancehall music are not
exactly the same as those of the emotive Negro spirituals Trumper
reveres. But it is a similar sense of "my people," a global African
consciousness, a joy in the rhythm of the word and the potency of the
beat that inspire youth throughout the Caribbean region and the
diaspora to respond to the pounding boom box of Jamaican popular
music and learn its compelling language.

Like George Lamming, Jamaican linguist Barbara Lalla seems to
apprehend the resonance of negritude and popular music. She argues in
Defining Jamaican Fiction: Marronage and the Discourse of Survival:

Nationalist discourse in the Caribbean has been deeply influenced by a
rhetoric of negritude, whose sources are as widespread (globally) as the

African diaspora itself. In Jamaica, oral discourse on negritude has been further influenced not only by oral traditions of folk culture but also, more recently, by those of black music culture. Jamaica has exported this culture through reggae music and has imported black American equivalents. Elsewhere in the Caribbean, current Jamaican dance-hall music (regularly known as Dansehall [*sic*]) has captivated youth and influenced their language. Parents commonly complain of being unable to understand a word of it, which may well account for its relative lack of restriction.[17]

But Lalla's reading of Jamaican dancehall music is decidedly ambivalent, echoing Ellis's *Talk Caribbean* definition of dancehall lyrics as unintelligible to adult ears. There is, as well, the insinuation that if the language were only understood, there would be the clear need for restriction/censure. Negritude in popular music seems not quite as respectable as its "folk culture" antecedents.

It is not surprising therefore that in the very next paragraph Lalla, like Rohlehr, reduces the body of Jamaican dancehall music to skeletal stereotype. Insistent reference to the discourse as "violent" is typical of this kind of simplistic reading of the dancehall. "Black poverty and exploitation" are minimized and become far less compelling signifiers of cultural meaning than is the generic "violence." There also seems to be an implicit reprimand of competitive performers who manage to be successful, despite their ghetto origins. But perhaps I am making too much of a hapless "however":

> In valorizing the ghetto, much Dansehall [*sic*] justifies violent resistance to black poverty and exploitation. At the same time, however, the competition between immensely successful performers expresses itself in terms of braggadocio and violent challenge. Oral sources of Dansehall and American rap perpetuate and strengthen stereotypes such as that of the black male as superhuman lover and in so doing entrench attitudes destructive to women. . . . Radical opposition to imperial discourse is thus, of itself, no longer avant-garde in the Caribbean but popular and even riddled with cliche.[18]

The very same could be said for not-so-radical opposition.

The Jamaican elite, as much as their Barbadian counterparts, fail to comprehend the unsettling language of youth. A classic example comes from the Jamaican television talk show *Perspective,* in a program on dancehall music aired on January 21, 2001. Entitled "Bu[r]n Dis, Bu[r]n Dat," the program focused on the inflammatory rhetoric of many DJs whose metaphorical language of violence is not always fully understood. In response to a video clip of the group TOK, Junes Hines, the show's moderator, claimed to understand the lyrics. Yet when pressed, she could not explain their meaning and clung desperately to the single word "shotta"—Jamaican slang for "gunman"—as evidence to support her assertion that the song is celebrating gun violence.

As it turns out, TOK's song is at least in part a derisory, cautionary tale *satirizing* wannabe shottas who, posing as the real thing, are forced to holler for protection when the big guns, like the eagle, start to fly. Far from simply celebrating gun violence in this song, TOK seem to be undermining the identity of gunman that is assumed as a sign of heroism and bravery in the urban jungles where black youth compete for respect. Like Ellis's "whore," Hines's "shotta" signifies a more complicated politics than these self-righteous authority figures would allow. And it all comes down to misunderstanding the language.

In sympathy with June Hines, I do concede that the speed of delivery of the DJ's lyrics does reduce intelligibility for all but the keenest ears. But failure to understand the lyrics is only one of a series of refusals in Jamaica to take Jamaican Creole seriously. The denial of the status of officially recognized national language for the mother tongue of the vast majority of Jamaicans is a perverse act of psychological brutality that attempts to undermine the self-confidence of monolingual Jamaican Creole speakers. This domestic politics of marginalization helps to explain the contempt for the Jamaican language outside the country—for example, among the Barbadian elite, as represented in the editorial outpourings of the *Advocate.* If we Jamaicans do not respect our own language, how can we expect others to valorize it?

In response to my critique of the "Vile Vocals" editorial, the *Advocate* published two other vile editorials, "Seek Quality: Chance in a UWI Review [*sic*]" and "Bad Product: Don't Import the Garbage." Here "garbage" refers explicitly to the Jamaican language:

> A University of the West Indies professor is expressing eagerness to return to Barbados to teach what she says is "Jamaican Creole." By "creole" she means an unstructured tongue masquerading as desirable communication outside her homeland.
>
> She omits to explain why her native Jamaica excludes baser aspects of that medium from radio and television broadcasts, but indicates these elements should be swallowed as some sort of elixir for Barbadian culture.
>
> Her diatribe last Sunday not only treats this island as an appropriate repository for her country's unwanted garbage, it further insults Barbadians by suggesting they are irrational and ignorant for objecting to its presence on our doorstep.[19]

It is instructive that, with its dependence on innuendo, the editorial conflates the Jamaican Creole language with lyrics composed in that language. The meaning of the phrase "baser aspects of that medium" is elusive. Is "medium" synonymous with "language"? And, if so, what constitutes the baseness of the language? The fact that it is a Creole language? And what precisely are the "aspects" and "elements" of this supposedly "unstructured tongue" that provoke such vacuous prose? But, perhaps, I ought not to look so hard for meaning in what is, after all, propagandist rhetoric masquerading as journalism.

It is true, as the editorial states, that "[l]yrics which Jamaica bans from its airwaves" are being played indiscriminately on the radio in Barbados—presumably because the meaning of these lyrics is not understood. If Bajans do not wish to sully their minds by learning Jamaican Creole, they would be well advised to employ translators to help them select the best of current Jamaican popular music: Luciano, Capleton,

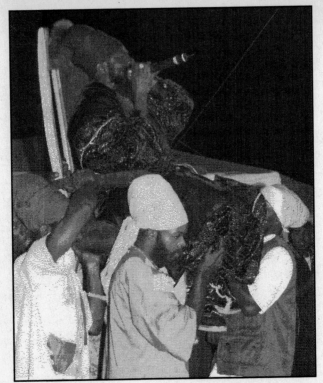

Capleton is brought to the stage like royalty at "Sting" 2002.
Photo: Ian Allen.

Sizzla, Anthony B, Buju Banton. But since much of the "conscious" dub music is coming from dreaded Rastafari—"the Caribbean's most embarrassing counter-culture" (to cite the "Vile Vocals" editorial), then Bajans end up hoisted on the petard of their combined ignorance and arrogance. The editorial glibly alleges that the lyrics of uncensored dub music "are having ruinous consequences in Barbados."[20] Where is the evidence? Where are the academic studies—not just talk-show hysteria—to prove the direct correlation between dub music on the radio and the rise in social problems in Barbados? Literate Bajans should be familiar with the *post hoc ergo propter hoc* fallacy: "after this therefore because of this." If Barbadian society appears to be falling apart after the advent of Jamaican dub music, this does not mean that dub music is the cause of the decline.

George Lamming's *In the Castle of My Skin* gives some very good clues to help us decipher the signs of social transformation in Barbados today. Lamming's schoolboys who daringly imagined the possibility of stoning the schoolteacher were so socialized to respect authority that no one could yield to temptation and cast the first stone. Similarly, those rebelling villagers who were tempted to stone the exploitative landlord Creighton daringly imagined the possibility but were so socialized to respect authority that no one could cast the first stone. Nowadays, the authority of the teachers-turned-politicians who betray the people is no longer blindly respected. And the Creightons of the world are no longer so sacred that they cannot be stoned.

Not surprisingly, the *Advocate* editorials do not tell the whole story of the wide-ranging Barbadian responses to Jamaican dancehall culture and, more specifically, to the representation of the issues addressed in the *Talk Caribbean* television program. The much more populist *Nation* newspaper had a decidedly liberal take on the topic. For example, there was an amusing cartoon in *Sunshine,* the *Nation*'s Sunday magazine of April 9, 2000, in which the following question is put in the mouth of Damon Chi-Anne Walker Foster, "almost 3 1/2 months old!": "I wonder if I gine ever [I'm ever going to] see a dub show at de Stadium."[18] This is a derisory reference to the fact that dub/dancehall shows were about to be banned at the National Stadium. The *Weekend Nation* of April 14, 2000, carried another subversive cartoon featuring a literal-minded customs officer interrogating a male visitor about the contents of his luggage: "Do you have any *explosives, firearms,* or dangerous goods like *dub CDs?*"[22]

In an insightful article, headlined "Dub's Not the Force of All Evil," Adonijah challenges the new policies, underscoring, the right-wing conservatism and shortsightedness of those imposing the ban:

There's a strange wind a-blowin'. And the wind is gathering force and threatening to blow away all in its path, innocent or otherwise.

What I'm referring to is the growing intolerance and right-wing perspective coming from sectors of Government and major players in society.

This has been expressed recently through the banning for the next 18 months of dub shows at the National Stadium and the statement that Customs will soon be checking on lyrics of recorded material passing through the ports of entry.

The dub ban is a worrying thing. First of all, as security forces in any metropolitan centre well know, people always need their escape valve. Taking it away is a dangerous thing, as it will only cause more pressure to build up.[23]

Adonijah also foregrounds intergenerational conflict and ideological dissonance within Barbados as factors motivating Bajan youth to pay attention to the "conscious" lyrics coming from the new wave of Rastafari DJs in Jamaica:

Secondly, ironically, the majority of the music performed at these shows at the stadium is positive and uplifting as far as the lyrics are concerned.

Anthony B, Sizzla, Capleton, Buju Banton, Jahmali, Luciano and *Yami Bolo*, for example, are all singers of very conscious lyrics, songs that help the youth to know their identity, something that their parents often did not and do not know.

Why rob the youth of this experience? Those on the outside may find it hard to accept but music of this kind acts as a positive influence on the youth, rather than a negative.[24]

In addition, Adonijah acknowledges the fact that indigenous Barbadian artists generate as much, if not more, social noise than their Jamaican counterparts. It is the failure of the Barbadian elite to hear this native noise and contemplate what it means that seems to motivate their simpleminded banning of the "foreign" overdub:

> Hasn't anyone noticed that there are seldom if ever any disturbances when artistes of this nature are performing?
>
> If security is a problem then there are certain Bajan bands that should be banned as well, for there is a history of disturbances when they perform. This is not a call for more banning but a call for more reason to be applied. Instead of looking for scapegoats, society has to come to grips with the fact that there are certain basic weaknesses in it.[25]

Speculation about the consequences of this ban on dangerously explosive dub music lyrics suggests that not only would homegrown varieties emerge in Barbados; even more alarming for the repressive elite is the frightening prospect that local social problems would not simply evaporate. Then a new scapegoat would have to be sent into the wilderness, bearing the sins of the people. Perhaps cricket. Since cricket incites such passion that outraged fans have been forced, on occasion, to throw bottles on the pitch, Barbados could then ban cricket, not just bottles.[26]

The liberal *Nation* gave wide coverage to the public lecture I delivered a few days after the *Talk Caribbean* television program. Entitled "Sweet & Sour Sauce: Sexual Politics in Jamaican Dancehall Culture," the lecture elaborated many of the issues raised on the television forum. Despite the hostility from on high to my academic work on Jamaican dancehall culture, I was heartened to discover that on the ground there is much support for the research in which I am engaged. I had been invited to give the public lecture by the Department of History at the University of the West Indies, Cave Hill, as part of series on gender and Caribbean history. The popular culture perspective I was bringing to the discourse was thus valorized.

After the lecture a concerned citizen asked me—and I paraphrase— why the Caribbean Broadcasting Corporation hadn't videotaped the talk. As all the others in the series of public lectures had been recorded, there was speculation that the controversial topic had made the cameras shy away. When I later checked with CBC I was assured that it was just "human error." Everywhere I went in the days following the *Talk Caribbean* broadcast I got positive vibrations—to cite Bob Marley. I presume that my detractors failed to voice their negative judgments in person. And there were many of these to be heard on the radio talk shows in the days following the lecture. Supportive comments at street level came from men and women, old and young. An older man in front of the Cave Shepherd department store observed that "the high-ups love calypso; dat is why deh ain't seh nothing bout it." A coconut vendor on Accra Beach asked, "Why deh don't talk bout di gun shooting [gun violence] on TV?" A watersports operator on the same stretch of beach said with conviction: "The problem is in the home, children having children." A beach sweeper called me out of the water to say, "I ain't see nothing wrong wid dub."

Positive vibes from all about: "I agree one hundred percent." "You too sweet." "Reggae is here to stay." "This is the woman who earned my respect." "You give a good account of you[r]self." "You gave them a hard time." A truck driver on Broad Street called: "Hey, Doc, enjoyed the show." A bright-eyed young woman for whom I hope I'm a good role model said: "I saw you on TV last night and you are one powerful woman." My favorite comment came from a charming older man: "Live here 'mongst us! You will do dat?" [Come and live here with us! Would you do that?] What I found most surprising was the meanspiritedness of the anonymous writer of the *Barbados Advocate*'s "Bad Product" editorial, who refused to concede that I could have received such positive feedback and thus questioned the authenticity of the responses. The clear insinuation was that I was lying—a remarkably desperate accusation: "With so little respect for basic etiquette as a guest in this country, the professor would have done very well indeed to have been paid the many compliments she glibly reproduced—verbatim—last Sunday; all apparently obtained without the aid of notebook or tape recorder."[27]

As it turns out, I did record, on a scrap of paper that I still have in my possession, many of the comments I received. I lost a fair number before it occurred to me that here was good, unsolicited data, given to me on a platter, that should not be discarded for the informality of its collection. One really ought not to look a gift horse in its mouth. Had I approached "respondents" with a tape recorder for a research project on popular Barbadian perceptions of Jamaican dancehall culture, I would not have received the spontaneous feedback I elicited. Nevertheless, this does not mean that a formal research project on the regional impact of Jamaican popular music ought not to be initiated. Hysteria and serendipity are no substitute for scholarship.

The exporting of Jamaican dancehall lyrics to Barbados and the wider eastern Caribbean reveals the problematic cultural politics of national identity in the so-called Anglophone Caribbean—despite the best efforts of CARICOM to consolidate an updated "federal" politics.[28] Contesting the viability of regional definitions of cultural identity, conservative nationalist discourses are asserting themselves with renewed authority. The censorious, purist rhetoric of the *Advocate*'s editorials and the surprising xenophobia of Curwen Best's declaration that Jamaican dancehall music is the quintessential Caribbean music of death exemplify this disturbing trend. Gordon Rohlehr's dismissal of both rap and Jamaican dancehall music as "songs of the skeleton" is also troubling. Furthermore, as local cultures in the Caribbean and elsewhere respond to the homogenizing imperative of the globalization epidemic, they are tempted to assert cultural autonomy as a self-protective vaccine. But whereas the elite in Barbados, for example, are terrified of the invasive "Trojan horse of a counter-culture" from Jamaica, the masses of the region's youths, both at home and in the Caribbean diaspora, embrace Jamaican dancehall music and its language as a celebratory discourse, asserting a shared identity of cultural affiliation.

EIGHT

Hip-hopping across Cultures

Reggae to Rap and Back

Nairobi's male elephants uncurl
their trumpets to heaven
Toot-Toot takes it up
in Havana
in Harlem

bridges of sound curve
through the pale rigging
of saxophone stops[1]

—Kamau Brathwaite

The African diasporic poet Kamau Brathwaite employs the resonant metaphor "bridges of sound" to evoke the substrate cultural ties that reconnect Africans on the continent to those who have survived the dismembering Middle Passage. The paradoxical construct, "bridges of sound," conjoins the ephemerality of aural sensation with the technological solidity of the built environment. This arresting metaphor affirms the creative potential of Africans in the diaspora to conjure knowledge systems out of nothing, as it were. Africans, taken away without tools, were able to rebuild material culture from the blueprint of knowledge carried in our collective heads. In long historical perspective, the Middle Passage thus functions like a musical bridge; it is a transitional passage connecting major sections of a musical composition. And that magnum opus is the survival song of generations of Africans who have endured the crossing.[2]

The poem "Jah" acknowledges the immediate excremental details of the Middle Passage and, simultaneously, celebrates the therapeutic power of the imagination to transform the real into the surreal. In a clever metaphorical slide, the rigging of the slave ship becomes the stops of the saxophone: "bridges of sound curve/ through the pale rigging/ of saxophone stops." This dislocating shift from the literal to the metaphorical may be read as a sign of the delirium of enslaved shipboard Africans trapped in a hallucinogenic trip of anticonquest. But the visionary turn from the rigging to the saxophone also can be conceived as a liberating trope of the processes of artistic creativity and aesthetic transformation.

Indeed, the poet as griot is moved to wonder if the drummer and the sound of the drum will continue to have potency after the debilitating sea change of the Middle Passage. The answer is a resounding yes. The capacity to make music anew does become quite literally the bridge of sound that rehumanizes enslaved people who have been cannibalized by history:

> the ship sails, slips on banana
> peel water, eating the dark men.
>
> Has the quick drummer nerves
> after the stink Sabbath's unleavened
> cries in the hot hull? From the top
> of the music, slack Bwana
> Columbus rides out of the jungle's den.
>
> With my blue note, my cracked note, full flatten-
> ed fifth, my ten bebop fingers, my black bottom'd strut, Panama

worksong, my cabin, my hut,

my new frigged-up soul and God's heaven

heaven, gonna walk all over God's heaven . . . (162-63)

Here Brathwaite names some of the musical forms that have emerged in the Americas—blues, jazz, work songs, and spirituals. The reference to Panama work songs acknowledges the labor-intensive project of constructing the canal and the role of music in sustaining the spirit in dehumanizing physical circumstances. The movement of Caribbean peoples to work on the canal made possible new processes of acculturation and reshaped old aesthetic forms. Indeed, "Panama" becomes a metaphor for the bridging of African diasporic cultures in the Americas. The canal, produced by the labor of so many remigrant African peoples, now separates continents and, simultaneously, joins the Atlantic to the Pacific Ocean—itself the locus of other African diasporas, both ancient and modern. Metaphorical bridges of sound span not only the Atlantic, but also overarch the many bodies of water that dis/connect African peoples dispersed across the globe: Nairobi to Havana, Havana to Harlem, Kingston to Panama.[3]

The eclectic music of the Panamanian American jazz pianist Danilo Perez exemplifies this aesthetic conjuncture. Fernando Gonzalez, the Arts and Culture writer of the *Miami Herald*, describes Perez's fourth CD this way:

In *Central Avenue*, Danilo Perez mixes blues, Middle Eastern-tinged melodies and the folk singing of rural Panama, conjures up Thelonius Monk playing 21st century *danzones*, sets Indian tablas next to Caribbean tumbadoras—and makes it all sound familiar. More than that, it sounds inevitable. Perhaps it is.

Perez is one of the many of us living in the United States on a moving border. It's a boundary crossed secretly, in plain sight, every day, many times a day, by necessity and chance. It's a crossing that turns us all into interpreters and translators, tour guides and *indocumentados*. We are respected shamans and brutes. Our images are a reflection in a funhouse mirror. Our language is a collection of found words and borrowed memories. We construct our past of what we create. We know who we are; it's just that we barely recognize ourselves sometimes. No wonder we can always tell which side of the border we are on, but not where home is. Of this, Perez creates a fresh new music that feels lived-in.[4]

There are so many diasporas within the Diaspora. The distinctive, neo-African musical forms that have emerged in the Caribbean, Latin America, North America, and the Pacific, for example, are vibrant testimony to the longevity and durability of sound musical bridges. Like jazz and the blues, more recent musics such as reggae, ragga/dancehall, and rap constitute sites of rebellion against the ubiquitous brutalization of African peoples. These new sounds of cultural warfare are contemporary manifestations of a long tradition of African diasporic hybridity and bricolage. The evolution of reggae in Jamaica illustrates this cross-fertilizing process.

Garth White, former research fellow in the International Reggae Studies Centre at the University of the West Indies, Mona, Jamaica, observes in an important 1982 monograph that mento, the indigenous folk music of Jamaica, absorbed influences from the Trinidad calypso and Cuban rumba. Indeed, White notes that: "the calypso and the mento were often so similar that the terms were often used interchangeably when referring to mento. At the same time, a number of differences can be observed between the two forms. Mento could be either fast or slow tempo, but it was usually slower than calypso, encouraging more sinuous, horizontal, pelvic movement in the dance."[5] Later, African American rhythm and blues influenced this already hybridized mento music, accelerating the process of transformation that resulted in ska. Ska decelerated into rock-steady, which, in turn, crescendoed into the dread beat of reggae. The latest incarnation of Jamaican popular music, variously known as dancehall, ragga, and dub, is an energetic fusion of electronically engineered *riddims* and traditional folk musical forms.

Jamaican-born radical poet and political activist Linton Kwesi Johnson, long resident in the United Kingdom, describes the new hybrid:

> With the discovery of digital recording, an extreme minimalism has emerged—in the music of people like Steelie and Cleevie [*sic*], for example. On one hand, this music is totally technological; on the other the rhythms are far more Jamaican: they're drawn from Etu, Pocomania, Kumina—African-based religious cults who provide the rhythms used by Shabba Ranks or Buju Banton. So despite the extent of the technology being used, the music is becoming even rootsier, with a resonance even for quite old listeners, because it echoes back to what they first heard in rural Jamaica.[6]

Many older listeners, however, simply cannot hear the reverberations. Instead, for them the "noise" of dancehall music engenders a sound clash with roots reggae music.

In an article entitled "First Reggae. Then Rap. Now it's Dancehall," Ben Mapp, writing in the *New York Times,* defines contemporary ragga/dancehall as "a cousin of both reggae and rap," noting that "[t]he dancehall D.J. is the equivalent of hip hop's M.C. or rapper, rhyming over the rhythms steeped in Jamaican patois."[7] The metaphor of blood relation is apt, but Mapp distorts the genealogy: "First Reggae. Then the old school Jamaican DJs. Then Rap. Now it's Dancehall." This bridging of reggae, ragga, and rap is the central preoccupation of this chapter, which is very much a work-in-progress.[8] In the fervent hope of absolution, I must confess that I am a neophyte in the communion of rap. I am not at all versed in its polysyllabic catechism.

Nevertheless, with the reckless presumption of the new convert, I dare to make a few generalizations about hip-hop culture and draw some parallels with Jamaica's dancehall culture, focusing on two clearly inter-connected areas: language and ideology. I do not provide details of the history of musical production across the related music genres. I leave that task to the musicologists who possess the requisite expertise. My formal training is in literary studies, and I am obviously moonlighting in foreign territory. In the circumstances I do believe that discretion is the better part of scholarship. I come to the project with an instinct for textual analysis and with a fascination for language and the movement of verbal meaning across cultural borders.

The naming of Jamaican popular music reveals complex ideological meanings. The words "reggae" and "ragga" share a common ragged etymology that denotes their identical urban ghetto origins in the concrete jungle of Kingston. The 1967 *Dictionary of Jamaican English* defines "reggae" as "a recently estab[lished] sp[elling] for *rege* (the basic sense of which is *ragged*—see *rege-rege* with possible ref[erence] to rag-time music (an early form of American jazz) but referring esp[ecially] to the slum origins of this music in Kingston." "Rege-rege" is defined first as "rags, ragged clothing"; its secondary meaning is "a quarrel, a row." The dictionary entry invites readers to compare "rege-rege" with "raga-raga," which is defined in the nominative as "old ragged clothes"; as adjective, it means "in rags, ragged"; and as verb, it means "to pull about, pull to pieces." In Jamaican Creole, there are a number words formed from the consonants *r* and *g/k* that share essentially the same meaning of ragged and connote disorder and deviation from the habits of respectability.[9] Words such as *tegereg* (related to the English tag-and-rag, meaning "of or belonging to the rabble") and *regjegz* (described in the *Dictionary of Jamaican English* as probably reduced from the English "rags and jags," "jags" meaning "rags and tatters"). A related word is *streggeh,* meaning "promiscuous woman."

Stephen Davis, author of *Reggae Bloodlines,* identifies the singer Toots Hibbert as the first to use the word "reggay" in the title of a song— the 1967 "Do the Reggay." The spelling variation confirms the fluidity of the word in this early period of formation. Davis reports his conversation with the singer on the etymology of "reggae" in this way: "I once asked Toots Hibbert, lead singer of the Maytals and composer of 'Do the Reggay,' to tell me what the word meant, and his answer is as satisfactory a definition of reggae as you're likely to get: 'Reggae means comin' from the people, y'know? Like a everyday thing. Like from the ghetto. From *majority*. Everyday thing that people use like food, we just put music to it and make a dance out of it. Reggae means *regular* people who are suffering, and don't have what they want.'"[10]

Hibbert's poetic reggae/regular word play emphasizes the everyday ordinariness of the basic survival strategies of "regular people who are suffering" and who use music and dance, like food, as essential nutrients for daily sustenance. In creolized Jamaican English "regular" would be pronounced "regla," thus reinforcing the echo of "reggae." The reggae/regla semantic shift deftly underscores the regulatory, safety-valve function of reggae music in Jamaican society. Without raga-raga music, the explosive class politics of stark deprivation versus vulgar privilege would detonate even more resoundingly than it now does. To indigenize Karl Marx's classic dictum that religion is the opium of the masses, I propose that in Jamaica reggae is the ganja of the *massive*.

The word "ragga" is an abbreviation of the English "ragamuffin," meaning "a ragged, dirty, disreputable man or boy"; also, "rough, beggarly, good-for-nothing, disorderly." In the contemporary Jamaican context, the semantic range of the word "ragamuffin" is widened to include the sense of glorified badmanism. There is thus enacted a process of subversion of the English meaning of the word whereby the outlaw condition of the ragamuffin is simultaneously transferred to and transformed in Jamaican usage. The Jamaican masses transgressively reclaim and celebrate the outlawry of ragamuffin-style dancehall music, which now bears the same stigma that reggae endured in its 1960s period of formation. Conversely, the Jamaican elite marginalizes both musics as outlaw sounds, though it must be conceded that, over time, the hard-hitting rebel music of a Bob Marley has become respectable: classical "roots and culture" reggae.

Jamaican music journalist Mandingo observes that the term "ragamuffin" and its variant, "ragamuffet," were first used in reggae in the 1978 tune "Ragamuffet," sung by Horace Andy and produced by Tappa Zukie for his

Star recording label. Mandingo says this on the provenance of the term "ragamuffin": "Shortened to 'Ragga' in England, it merely means those person[s] whom Jkans [Jamaicans] used to call Rudies, Rebels, Spengs, or Soldiers. The names simply describe rebellious youths who managed to survive and flourish. . . ."[11] Mandingo emphasizes the inventiveness of these ragamuffin youths who defy the eurocentric conventions of middle-class respectability in Jamaica: "These Ragamuffins have always clung to their grassroots culture and have created and continued to create new music, dance and styles that influence and inspire the rest of the world. There is positive and negative in everything and reggae dancehall Raga-muffin is no exception!"[12] The very same could be said of rap music, with its similar origins in New York's concrete jungle.

In the various versions of the story of rap that I've reviewed, there is a remarkable coherence of theme. All of the narratives define a confluence of forces that produce the new music. The recurring themes are (1) displace-ment, (2) cultural alienation, (3) technological inventiveness, (4) verbal virtuosity, and (5) gender politics. Freelance journalist Raquel Rivera observes that "hip hop was intimately related to the socioeconomic and political realities of the time. The social conditions and economic pros-pects for young people living in poor urban communities during the 1960s and 1970s were appalling. African Americans and Puerto Ricans living in New York, in particular, shared similar conditions and, quite often, the same workplaces and dilapidated neighborhoods, and were served by the same decaying schools and hospitals. As Bronx DJ, producer and MC KMX-Assault explains of Blacks and Puerto Ricans in New York during the 1960s and 1970s: 'You lived next door; you shared the same cock-roaches.'"[13]

In this same period, the South Bronx home of rap was the site of radical social and spatial transformation precipitated by the construction of the Cross-Bronx Expressway, begun in 1959. Tricia Rose cites Marshall Berman's account of the devastating impact of construction work: "Miles of streets alongside the road were choked with dust and fumes and deafening noise. . . . Apartment houses that had been settled and stable for over twenty years emptied out, often virtually overnight; large and impoverished black and Hispanic families, fleeing even worse slums, were moved wholesale, often under the auspices of the Welfare Department, which even paid inflated rents, spreading panic and accelerating flight. . . . Thus depopulated, economically depleted, emotionally shattered, the Bronx was ripe for all the dreaded spirals of urban blight."[14]

The dust, fumes, and noise of the invasive expressway are sensational manifestations of class politics. In this ideological race/class/culture sound clash the powerful are free to impose their deafening noise on the powerless. In the battle for the control of "public" space, the poor usually lose. Displacement exacerbates the cultural alienation of the politically marginalized. The French philosopher Jacques Attali has defined music as "the organization of noise."[15] This brilliant aphorism encodes a sophisticated understanding of the complex ways in which the power to organize noise is appropriated differently in different cultures. Black youths in the destabilized South Bronx used their skills in electronics to reorganize the dissonance in their environment. They learned to make music out of social noise.

The metaphor of noise recurs in the vocabulary of rap. The *A 2 Z: The Book of Rap and Hip-Hop Slang* defines noise as "the sound or phenomenon of rap."[16] The citation selected to illustrate the entry on noise is a quote from Chuck D: "People try to come up with intellectual reasons for the noise, and it ain't nothing intellectual."[17] The reputed anti-intellectualism of the noise is decidedly an intellectual issue. Indeed, Chuck D himself elaborates a politics of noise in a brilliant television interview: "What we saying can also be viewed as noise, irritating, oh no stop it, turn it off. And, ahm, we're gonna bring it regardless. So we're gonna be too black and too strong and just deal with whatever comes down the line."[18]

The politics of exclusion and inclusion reverberate in rap. Insiders understand the noise. They participate in a communicative field that gives meaning to the dissonant pain of everyday survival. Outsiders dismiss as mere "noise" the guttural sounds that affirm the African American's right to speech in the public sphere. The recuperation of "noise" as a positive affirmation of the politics of inclusion is an excellent example of the way in which African American speech subverts the lexicon of American English to articulate in-group identity. Linguist Geneva Smitherman locates hip-hop discourse within the broader context of subversive African American speech practices: "Today Hip Hoppers call it *flippin the script*. . . . This is a process much more profound than the creation of mere 'slang.' From its origin as a counter language, flippin the script has resulted in a coded Black Semantics, available only to Africans in America. This accounts for the fact that when a term crosses over and gains linguistic currency in the EAL [European American English] world AAL [African American Language] speakers generate a new term to take its place."[19]

The hip-hop metaphor of flippin the script suggests the autonomy of authorship, the creative capacity of the artist to rewrite the submissive script of compliant silence that has been imposed on African Americans. This cry for equal rights and justice is the universal noise of the ghetto. For example, the Fugees, Haitian American refugee rappers, appropriate Bob Marley's "No Woman, No Cry," transforming this song of consolation into "a dedication to all the refugees worldwide."[20] Forced to become refugees, the dislocated have had to endure "the pain of losing family." In their recontexualization of Marley's lyrics, the Fugees reconfigure the boundaries of his grief, widening the family of shared suffering and mutual consolation.

Marley's "government yard in Trench Town" becomes the Fugees' "government yard in Brooklyn" and "project yard in Jersey." There, in Brooklyn, they observe the "crookedness as it mingle with the good people." Marley's "hypocrites" who mingle with the good people become the Fugees' generic "crookedness." This revision evokes the hip-hop *signifyin* on Brooklyn as "Crooklyn." Marley's poignant reference to Georgie lighting ghetto fires gets a new urban twist of "drive-by" violence in the Fugees' version: "Little Georgie would make the fire light/ As stolen cars pass through the night." In an understandable gesture of inclusion, the Fugees draw even the fugitive gunman into the circle of refugees: "The gunman's in the house tonight/ But everything's gonna be alright." Marley's culture-specific references assume new diasporic meanings as they cross borders.

Rap, like reggae, is the noise of remembering. And technological inventiveness does amplify the noise—the verbal virtuosity—of the dispersed African community. Music critic David Toop has traced the convoluted genealogy of rap right back across the Middle Passage to West Africa: "Rap's forebears stretch back through disco, street funk, radio DJs, Bo Diddley, the bebop singers, Cab Calloway, Pigmeat Markham, the tap dancers and comics, The Last Poets, Gil Scott-Heron, Muhammad Ali, acappella and doo-wop groups, ring games, skip-rope rhymes, prison and army toasts, signifying and the dozens, all the way to the griots of Nigeria and the Gambia."[21]

Toop also acknowledges the immediate influence of Caribbean music in catalyzing the processes of hybridization that erupted as rap in late 1970s' urban Black America, underscoring the role of Caribbean migration into New York and the resulting acculturation. For example, the parents of hip-hop DJ Grandmaster Flash migrated from Barbados, and his father was a connoisseur of both American and Caribbean music.

Toop confirms the fundamental influence of Jamaican sound system technology on the evolution of rap. Reggae itself did not cross over widely into Black American culture in the 1970s, but its sound system mode of transmission did. The migrant Jamaican Clive Campbell, aka Kool DJ Herc, brought the noise to the Bronx. Toop observes that: ". . . it was the 'monstruous' [*sic*] sound system of Kool DJ Herc which dominated hip hop in its formative days. Herc came from Kingston, Jamaica, in 1967, when the toasting or DJ style of his own country was fairly new. Giant speaker boxes were essential in the competitive world of Jamaican sound systems (sound system battles were and still are central to the reggae scene) and Herc murdered the Bronx opposition with his volume and shattering frequency range."[22]

Sociologist Dick Hebdige documents Herc's inventiveness in responding to his audience's rejection of reggae. Herc "began talking over the Latin-tinged funk that he knew *would* appeal. To start with he merely dropped in snatches of street slang, like the very first toaster djs who worked for Coxsone Dodd's system in the 1950s."[23] Herc isolated the particular organization of noise that would capture the imagination of his predominantly African American audience; this was the instrumental break. Hebdige notes, "The lead guitar or bass riff sequence of drumming that he wanted might last only fifteen seconds. Rather than play the whole record straight through he would play this same part several times over, cutting from one record deck to the other as he talked through the microphone."[24]

Hebdige gives a classic example of the recycling of diasporic sound in his account of Herc's resuscitation of the song "Apache," released in 1974 and performed by the Jamaican disco group, the Incredible Bongo Band. The song, "written for the Shadows, Cliff Richard's backing group, in 1974 . . . had been 'covered' by an American group called The Ventures, who had a minor hit with it in the States."[25] The Jamaican group "used conga drums instead of the standard pop music drum kit. And they laid more stress on the percussion. Thanks to Kool Herc, *Apache* could be heard all over the Bronx in 1975."[26] But it was and wasn't "Apache." Herc's inventiveness had transformed the instrumental break into a bridge of sound that made the Jamaican disco version of an American hit acceptable to African American ears; in the process, he created an entirely new musical genre.

Like African American language, Jamaican Creole, the devalorized, hybrid language created by African peoples in Jamaica, is the preferred medium for rewriting and voicing-over the flipped script of cultural autonomy. The reggae singers and ragga DJs of Jamaica and its diasporas in the Caribbean, Africa, the Pacific, North and South America, and Europe draw on a tradition of resistance that is encoded in the language of Jamaican popular culture. Conservative, eurocentric (mis)conceptions of Jamaican as "broken," "bad," "corrupt" English deconstruct the language as pathology, a degeneration of the idealized "Queen's English." Conversely, metaphors of freedom in the popular imagination—for example, *"bruck out inna patwa"*—evoke the liberating discourse of breaking out of the prison of English grammar. Emancipating themselves from the inhibiting language of neocolonial schooling, the DJs, even more so than the early reggae singers, reclaim the power to speak authoritatively in their native language, with full knowledge of all its idiosyncrasies and creative possibilities.

Not surprisingly, in the crossing over of reggae, ragga, and rap in the U.S. East Coast, some Jamaican words have made their way into the vocabulary of hip-hop. And a few hip-hop terms have migrated into Jamaican dancehall culture. Two examples of hip-hop crossovers are "chronic," a particularly strong strain of ganja, and the honorific "G" for gangsta.[27] *A 2 Z: The Book of Rap and Hip-Hop Slang* has twelve entries that are identified as of Jamaican origin. These constitute a mere 0.6 percent of the dictionary's approximately two thousand entries. Below is a list of these words with their assigned meanings, some of which are not accurate translations of the Jamaican:

chatting: rapping

culture: serious affirmative lyrics of an historical or social nature

dancehall: contemporary reggae music or the club where it is played

dibi dibi: 1. n. a promiscuous female 2. adj. vulnerable or weak

gal pinkney[28]: an attractive female

level the vibes: to calm down the atmosphere in a music club or elsewhere

natty or natty dread: admirable

rewind: 1. vb. a DJ backspinning a record to the beginning 2. n. what an approving crowd shouts to the DJ

rude boy: n. and adj.: like ragamuffin; the West Indian equivalent of gangsta, gangsta rap music, gangsta-style clothes, and street slang

selecta: a DJ who favors reggae music

slackness: lyrics that are sexual rather than socially significant

sound boy: an MC, DJ, or other fixture at a reggae club

Nine additional entries, although not identified as of Jamaican origin, probably are: "dreads" is defined as "characteristic braided hair of Jamaican Rastafarians." Two entries point to the hybrid identities that are created in the movement between Jamaica and the United States: "Jafakein"—"false Jamaican"—and "Jamericans"—"American-born people with Jamaican parents." There is also the word "Jamdown," meaning "Jamaica." Surprisingly, "ragamuffin," in its culture-specific Jamaican sense of glorified badness, is not identified as Jamaican, although the definition clearly acknowledges its Jamaican roots: "roughneck or gangsta-style West Indian reggae music, or the 'rude boy' Jamaican equivalent of gangstas, gangsta fashion and street slang." Similarly, "toastin" ("dissing or boasting in a story, rhyming verbal format preceding rap") is not identified as Jamaican, although the secondary meaning assigned it, "rhyming verbal format preceding rap," may be read as an allusion to the Jamaican art form imported by Kool DJ Herc. "Pom-pom" ("vagina") with the variant spelling "pum-pum" and "pum-pum shorts" is not identified as Jamaican. Neither is "poonani" ("vagina"), which does have African American variants—"poontang" and "pootanany."[29]

Failure to assign Jamaican origin to these questionable entries may be simply an error on the part of the compilers. More profoundly, it may signify the depth of penetration of Jamaican words into hip-hop culture. The Jamaican origin is effaced and words become naturalized like their Jamerican carriers. A classic example of this process is the emergence of the quintessential hip-hop word "b-boy," not to be confused with the Jamaican "batty-bwoy," meaning "homosexual." Geneva Smitherman defines "b-boy" as:

A male follower of HIP HOP. Originally (in the Bronx and Harlem in the 1970s) B-boys referred to BROTHAS who would regularly "break" out into a dance movement to the DJ's scratching of a record. The term *B-boy* is believed to have been coined by the entertainer Kool DJ Herc. "Break" dancing, a rhythmic, intense type of dancing with twirls, turns, and intricate, fancy steps, is rooted in African and Caribbean dance movements.[30]

In the "Looking for the Perfect Beat" video, KRS One describes the process of semantic widening of the term "b-boy," which now includes a specifically Jamaican "hardcore" meaning:

Throughout the years a b-boy became a "bad bwoy" [laughs] on another level because the term "b-boy" began to go to everybody in the hip-hop community that felt as though that in order to maintain strength in the community we had to show ourselves as hardcore. And a lot of us—the half that was trying to survive—got caught up in the "bad bwoy" life.[31]

The cross-cultural reach of the word "poonani" confirms the magnetic pull of this female body part in the predominantly homosocial world of both rap and ragga music production. Clad—or, more accurately, barely clad—in pum-pum shorts, female genitalia figure frontally in the discourse of both ragga and rap. Gyrating female bodies are the standard visual vocabulary of both rap and dancehall videos. It is this overexposure of the more often brown than Black female body that accounts, in part, for the characterization of both rap and ragga as irredeemably misogynist. But, as I argue in chapter 3, women's unrestrained participation in dancehall culture as fans, performers, producers, and managers may signify not so much their mindless complicity in subjugation to dominating male discourses as their self-conscious celebration of the power of female sexuality to command submissive male attention. I do concede that the line between celebration and exploitation of the Black female body is rather thin, as thin as some of the fashionable garments sported by women in the dancehall.

In both African American hip-hop and Jamaican dancehall culture there appears to be an unresolved contradiction between "slackness" and

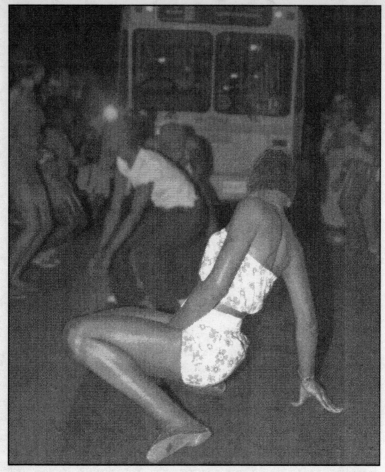

Passa Passa in downtown Kingston is where buses and dancers meet on the street.
Photo: Carlington Wilmot.

"culture." These Jamaican words, which have migrated into the vocabulary of rap, denote two ideological extremes. "Culture" connotes lyrics
that have a social and political "message." These lyrics usually decry the
dehumanizing conditions in which many African diasporic communities
eke out an existence. Racism, in particular, is the focus of many "culture"
lyrics. The names of rap groups such as Public Enemy articulate the

oppositional stance that many rappers assume in relation to the dominant political order. In Jamaican dancehall culture issues of race and class do surface in "conscious lyrics." Buju Banton's *'Til Shiloh* exemplifies the trend toward old-style message music of the "roots and culture" variety.[32]

Conversely, "slackness" is a gendered political space in which men assume absolute power in their sexual relations with women. This, too, is "message" music. Women become "bitches" and "(w)ho(re)s" and appear to be objectified in an overwhelmingly misogynist and verbally violent discourse. West Coast gangsta rap has decided affinities with Jamaican dancehall gun lyrics. The gun-toting heroes and antiheroes of countless Hollywood westerns and gangster flicks are alive and well in the macho world of Black popular music lyrics. This aggressive verbalization of male dominance may, in fact, be the impotent manifestation of a diminished masculinity seeking to exercise control in the only way it can. The recurring metaphor of the penis as gun in both rap and ragga lyrics is instructive.

Controversial African American psychiatrist Frances Cress Wesling argues in a provocative essay, "Guns as Symbols," that the gun as metaphorical phallus bears the weight of white male sexual inadequacy in relation to Black males:

> The gun became not only the weapon, the developed technology to ensure white genetic survival, but it also became the symbolic white penis. Thus it is no accident that white males often refer to one another as 'son of a gun.' . . . This phrase deprecates the white male genital apparatus that "fathers" white people. . . . It says instead that the white male prefers the gun to be his phallus and the phallus of his father. The gun then becomes the desired all-powerful phallus of the white male, which he conceives of as being the equalizer to the phallus of Black and non-white males.[33]

This inflammatory reading of the gun as symbolic white phallus raises the problematic issue of Black male appropriation of the deadly insecurities of white males. In Black neighborhoods—the hood—the Black man's literal gun is pointed more often at other Black males than at white males. Subversive hierarchies of impotence become established when Black men use the gun to assert authority over men and women within their own community. But Black women do not always passively accept the threat of Black male violation of their person. Female rappers like Queen Latifah and female DJs like Lady Saw give as much as they get. They assume the power to give back-chat. Flipping the script, they contest the negative roles assigned them, even as they seem to submit to stereotype.

Cheryl Keyes concludes her illuminating article "'We're More than a Novelty, Boys': Strategies of Female Rappers in the Rap Music Tradition," with the following insight:

> There still exists among women of rap a conscious need to maintain a sense of womanliness and "female respectability that is the ideal of feminine face" in this male-dominated tradition. Some have chosen to utilize the term *ladies* without having to justify their doing so, as in Queen Latifah's rap "Ladies First," while others like Yo-Yo, have started such organizations as the Intelligent Black Women's Coalition (I.B.W.C.) in response to the rap industry's ongoing sexism, including misogynist lyrics. In general, women express through the rap medium their personal feelings about female and male relationships, but more important, they speak for the empowerment of women. Although acceptance and recognition are crucial to contemporary women of rap, they want to be regarded as more than just a novelty.[34]

Reggae, rap, and ragga originate in a complex ideological space in which identity is continually contested; binaries such as "insider" and "outsider," "native" and "foreigner," "*wi*" and "*dem*" are subject to constant revision. Profound issues of race, class, and gender are represented in the noisy discourse of African diasporic popular music. In the words of Chuck D, "Rap music makes up for its lack of melody with its sense of reminder."[35] Ragga, too often dismissed as noise, not music, tells its own story of cultural remembering. Similarly, the disturbing lyrics of "roots and culture" reggae sing of displacement, cultural alienation, and the search for home in the diaspora. Chuck D's ominous sense of reminder is the bridge of sound that connects reggae, rap, and ragga to their multivocal, Middle Passage antecedents.

NINE

"Mix Up the Indian with All the Patwa"

Rajamuffin Sounds in "Cool" Britannia

The international dispersal of Jamaican dancehall culture, as the music first accompanies migrant Jamaicans to Britain and North America and then becomes more broadly incorporated into the global economy of the multinational entertainment industry, raises complex ideological issues of "authenticity," "identity," and "diaspora politics." As reggae/ragga goes "mainstream," much remains of the (con)tributary Jamaican cultural values. But these are constantly swirling in the cross-currents that bear the music along. A classic example of these processes of interculturation is the emergence of DJ Apache Indian (Steve Kapur), in Birmingham, England. His career illustrates, as well, the necessary adaptation of this potent Jamaican dancehall culture to accommodate local needs in its global spread.

Jamaican popular culture is an important site of resistance to, and co-optation by, the insatiable demands of capitalist consumerism. Stuart Hall, the Jamaican-born don of British Cultural Studies, underscores the inherent contradictions of the mass marketing of popular culture. Resistance to

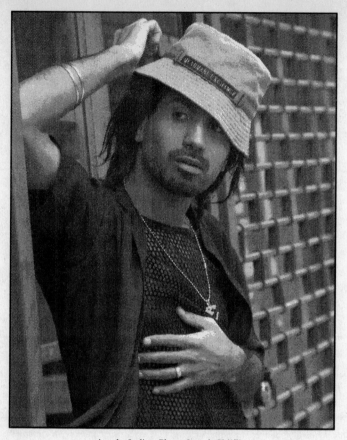

Apache Indian. Photo: Joseph Chielli.

subordination is a primary function of localized popular culture; but that "resistance" often is undermined by complicity with the countervailing economic imperatives of the global market:

> The role of the "popular" in popular culture is to fix the authenticity of popular forms, rooting them in the experiences of popular communities from which they draw their strength, allowing us to see them as expressive

of a particular subordinate social life that resists its being constantly made over as low and outside.

However, as popular culture has historically become the dominant form of global culture, so it is at the same time the scene, *par excellence,* of commodification, of the industries where culture enters directly into the circuits of a dominant technology—the circuits of power and capital. It is the space of homogenization where stereotyping and the formulaic mercilessly process the material and experiences it draws into its web, where control over narratives and representations passes into the hands of the established cultural bureaucracies, sometimes without a murmur. It is rooted in popular experience and available for expropriation at one and the same time.[1]

How is Apache Indian's appropriation of the language and persona of the generic Jamaican dancehall DJ to be read? As an interloper's mercilessly formulaic reprocessing of a stereotypical diasporic Jamaican politics of resistance? Or as an articulate, empathetic translation into another idiom of Apache Indian's own experience as a multilingual, border-crossing urban youth? Or both? Anticipating these skeptical questions, the DJ unambiguously declares:

Nough a [lots of] dem a talk bout me a coolie
And from there so now them want take liberty
Them can't realise, no, them just can't see
That from me come me no dis nobody.
Me a push reggae music to a different body
A next nation and a next country
And from fe me style people dem a ask me
About the one call Shabba and the one called Cutty
And about Supercat and Sweetie Irie
But me no mind how a bwoy no[w] him want dis me
Ca me walk and a talk with the almighty[2]

"Me a push reggae music to a different body/ A next nation and a next country": The use of both "nation" and "country" may, at first, be dismissed as a mere redundancy, a consequence of the DJ's need to extend the metrical line and accommodate the rhyme. But especially in a context such as the United Kingdom, "nation" and "country" are *not* synonymous. "Nation," with its emotive resonances of shared histories and cultural traditions, is a category that deliberately excludes many citizens, both migrant and native born, from any fundamental(ist) identification with their country of residence. Indeed, Apache Indian's "nation" encompasses an expansive body of South Asian/West Indian diasporic communities and others far beyond his country of birth. To these new global audiences—bodies, nations, and countries—the DJ offers himself as an unapologetic interpreter of Jamaican dancehall culture. In that process of interpretation he redefines the borders of his community.

Birmingham, the hometown of Apache Indian, is a major center of Caribbean and South Asian migration to Britain. A 1959 letter, written by Councillor Collett and published in the *Birmingham Evening Mail*, illustrates the "welcome" most immigrants could be expected to receive from the reluctant "host" society. This remarkably frank letter, with its novel recommendation of a limited license to guarantee the immigrant's good behavior, is reproduced in a 1967 book, *Race, Community, and Conflict: A Study of Sparkbrook*, coauthored by the sociologists John Rex and Robert Moore:

> How much longer have we Englishmen to tolerate the overt propaganda urging us to love the coloured immigrant who comes in peace and humility and ends by being the arrogant boss. For proof speak to or visit the white people living under a coloured landlord. On Monday a T.V. programme showed how a coloured man suffered when he came to live amongst us. He was expected to do the menial jobs and why shouldn't he? Few if any are capable of doing a skilled job and they could, of course, return home. But do they? Not on your life! Whether they be intellectual or not, they stay on,

hoping to wear us down with the old theme "love they neighbour." Only
good coloured immigrants should be allowed to come here, good in morals
and health, and they should be licensed so that their good behaviour and
limitation is guaranteed.[3]

The Sparkbrook study arose from the 1963 project, the Survey of
Race Relations in Britain, which was "concerned with the implications for
British Society of the presence of a substantial number of Commonwealth
immigrants."[4] Funded by the Nuffield Foundation, the survey was "conducted under the auspices of the Institute of Race Relations, an unofficial
and nonpolitical body, founded in England in 1958 to encourage and
facilitate the study of the relations between races everywhere."[5] According
to John Rex and Sally Tomlinson in a later book, Sparkbrook had been
selected "as a representative immigrant area in the twilight zone or the zone
of transition."[6]

By contrast, the Handsworth district was then seen as a "characteristically West Indian area as compared with Sparkbrook which was mixed,
but Pakistani and Irish dominated."[7] But within a few years the demogra-
phy of Handsworth was transformed. Rex and Tomlinson report, "There
were actually 9,116 Asian-born (principally Indian) residents in the four
wards of Sandwell, Handsworth, Soho and Newton (which in popular
usage are collectively referred to as Handsworth) as against 8,880 West
Indians, according to the 1971 census, suggesting a roughly equal West
Indian and Indian presence."[8] It is in Handsworth that Apache Indian was
born. This hybrid cultural space engenders a paradoxical politics of
alienation from and identification with the cultural "other."

George Lipsitz, professor of ethnic studies at the University of
California, San Diego, locates Apache Indian thus: "In 1993, audiences
around the world began hearing the music of an artist calling himself
'Apache Indian.' Because of his stage name and the title of his first album,
No Reservations, some speculated that he might be an American Indian.
But his music had the hard edge of Jamaican raggamuffin dance-hall rap,

suggesting that he might be West Indian. In fact, Apache Indian turned out to be Steve Kapur, a former welder from Handsworth in England whose parents were Punjabi immigrants from the southwest Asian nation of India."[9] In the Jamaican mento tune, "Soldering a wa di young gyal waan," [soldering is what the young girls want], soldering is a metaphor for the heat of sexual intercourse. Thus Apache Indian's former trade as welder seems a most appropriate apprenticeship for his present career as rajamuffin DJ.

Lipsitz highlights the importance of Apache's Handsworth origins in shaping the diverse musical elements that have been cut and mixed to produce the DJ's distinctive multiculti sound:

> Kapur grew up in the same racially-mixed neighbourhood that produced the inter-racial reggae band UB40 [and the all black Steel Pulse of "Handsworth Revolution" fame], and took his stage name in honor of his idol, the West Indian artist Wild Apache, aka Super Cat, both because Kapur admired his music and because Wild Apache himself included Caribbean East Indians among his ancestors.
>
> Apache Indian's music mixes hip-hop, reggae and Anglo-American pop styles with the Asian-Indian dance music bhangra, leading some commentators to call his music bhangramuffin. "I grew up in a very multicultural space," he explains, "where you can't get away from the reggae sound, and as an Asian, you can't get away from the bhangra sound, and living in this country, you can't get away from pop. All these flavors just came out."[10]

Michael Peter Smith, professor of community studies and development at the University of California, Davis, argues that among the many sociocultural, political, and economic forces that motivate transnational migration, a prime mover is "the globalization of mass communications, including television, film, video and music, which scatter the symbolic ingredients of 'imagined lives' and modes of self-empowerment at the 'core' to even the remotest of peripheral hinterlands."[11] But the transnational flow of media images is not one way, from imagined "core" to disempowered "periphery," as conventionally conceived. In the case of the dispersal of reggae, the periphery/core locution is itself dislocated. Hardcore Jamaican cultural values are exported globally in the music and exert a powerful influence on the host society.

Despite the limitations of Smith's static model of unidirectional cultural flows, he is nevertheless accurate in his assessment of the end result of these waves of cultural admixture: "Taken together, these transnational processes have reconstituted the sociocultural landscape and eroded the boundary-setting capacities of the nation-state. They have rendered problematic representations of the interplay between the state and civil society premised on clear distinctions between inside and outside, citizen and alien, self and other."[12] In transnational perspective, "the Caribbean" can no longer be contained within the conventional boundaries of the geo/logical nation-state. Apache Indian's Birmingham is, in many ways, a Caribbean city, a Jamaican city—subject to the media-colonizing power of Jamaican popular culture.

The often-unwelcome influx of immigrants from the former colonies into the British mainstream has irredeemably "polluted" the stream. Indeed, contemporary "mainstream" popular culture in postcolonial Britain is so contaminated that the nation has been forced to make a virtue of miscegenation. The Tony Blair revisioning of "Rule Britannia" as "Cool Britannia" is an acknowledgment—however facile—of a cultural style that is no longer monochromatic. The culture of the colonized, which was once seen purely as contaminant, is now celebrated in the new, skin-deep fiction of cool "multiculti" Britain. And it is only skin-deep, as illustrated in this photo caption published in the Jamaican *Gleaner:* "Designer Andrew Walsh is seen with his controversial black granite statue of Diana, Princess of Wales in this file picture May 19, 2000. The black statue of the late Princess Diana is now on display in a bus station in the English town of Walsall, after plans to install it in the town's new art gallery were scrapped by the local council because her family disapproved of the sculpture."[13] Blair's Britannia may be "cool," but in some quarters there is frosty resistance to alternative images of Britain as anything but pearly white.

Steel Pulse's "Roller Skates" articulates the problematic politics of transcultural/racial identification in an "uncool" Britannia whose rulers certainly know how to market "hot" merchandise. A Black man on roller skates, hanging out on the corner and enjoying his music, blasting from his radio, is approached by "this guy in his flashy car/ In his mouth a big cigar."[14] Ostensibly seeking directions, the criminal fat cat distracts the attention of the man, grabs his radio, and makes a dash for it. A police alert is sounded, and the thief is soon located.[15] Jamaican folklorist and poet Louise Bennett anticipates such acts of cultural appropriation in her humorous poem "Colonisation in Reverse." There she uses the subversive image of history turned upside down to represent the cultural dynamics of the Jamaicanization of English folkways:

> What a islan! What a people!
> Man an woman, ole an young
> Jussa pack [are just packing] dem bag and baggage
> An tun [and turning] history upside dung![16]

The musical "bag an baggage" of the rag-bag Jamaican yardies is quickly picked up, unpacked, and appropriated, raggamuffin style.

The crossover politics of transethnic acculturation in "Black" Britain is exemplified in the emergence of new lexical items such as *"rajamuffin"/ "raggastani"* and in the confluence of popular cultural formations to which these terms apply. In the structurally adjusted rag-bag word "rajamuffin," the English morpheme "rag" is replaced by the Hindi word "raj." Similarly, "raggastani" fuses "stan," the Hindi word for "place of origin," with the Jamaican abbreviation of "ragamuffin." Both "rajamuffin" and "raggastani" thus encode complex processes of cross-cultural accommodation in Black

Britain where "Black" signifies all "nonwhite" peoples, not only Africans—whether immediately from the continent or hyphenated over time and space.

But ethnic distinctions are nevertheless observed when this becomes politically expedient. The September 19, 1995, issue of *The Guardian* featured a "special investigation" on "violence in Britain." Vivek Chaudhury's article, which seeks to answer the question "Are we about to witness an explosion in Asian Crime?" is headlined "Enter the Rajamuffins." The opening paragraph explicitly criminalizes Jamaican yardies, defining them as the stylish name brand of which their emergent Asian counterparts are a clever *raja* rip-off:

> While the *yardie* has become synonymous with black crime, the *rajamuffin* is waiting to explode on to our streets, some would have us believe. The term is a tongue-in-cheek plagiarism of raggamuffin, the stylish, street-wise Jamaican youngsters with a fondness for crime who have influenced an entire urban culture in Britain. The rajamuffin is his Asian equivalent and he represents a departure from the stereotype of the law-abiding Asian who is more likely to be a victim of crime than a perpetrator.[17]

One suspects that many of Mr. Chaudhury's "Jamaican youngsters" are born in Britain. Indeed, Tony Thompson notes in an article in that same *Guardian* special investigation on crime that:

> So enduring is this association [of "Jamaican"] with extreme violence, and the dubious form of respect that it brings, that many young blacks from a variety of ethnic origins play up their own, usually non-existent, links with the Yardies in order to reinforce their reputations. There have even been cases of Nigerian and Ghanaian drug dealers attempting to affect Jamaican accents in order to enhance their status.[18]

Here "Jamaican" signifies not so much literal nationality as transgressive, transnational cultural style—Raggastani/rajamuffin style. Thompson's article opens with a melodramatic question: "How has a ramshackle criminal syndicate from Jamaica carved out a brutal reputation for fearsome violence?"[19] Perhaps the only right answer is another question: from Jamaica?

In the quintessentially "Black British" novel, *White Teeth,* Zadie Smith gives a brilliant reading of the genealogy of rajamuffin/raggastani youth in Britain, foregrounding the South Asian interculturation within the subculture:

> It was a new breed, just recently joining the ranks of the other street crews: Becks, B-boys, Indie kids, wide-boys, ravers, rudeboys, Acidheads, Sharons, Tracies, Kevs, Nation Brothers, Raggas, and Pakis; manifesting itself as a kind of cultural mongrel of the last three categories. Raggastanis spoke a strange mix of Jamaican patois, Bengali, Gujurati, and English. Their ethos, their manifesto, if it could be called that, was equally a hybrid thing: Allah *featured,* but more as a collective big brother than a supreme being, a hard-as-fuck *geezer* who would fight in their corner if necessary; kung fu and the works of Bruce Lee were also central to the philosophy; added to this was a smattering of Black Power (as embodied by the album *Fear of a Black Planet,* Public Enemy); but mainly their mission was to put the Invincible back in Indian, the Bad-aaaass back in Bengali, the P-Funk back in Pakistani.[20]

Taken out of the exclusively criminal context in which Chaudhury locates it, rajamuffin/raggastani discourse encodes the broader processes of Black-on-Black acculturation in Britain engendering, for example, hybrid popular music forms like bhangramuffin, also known as bhangraragga. In yet another *Guardian* story headlined "Intriguing Outcastes," which features the cleverly named Asian club and record label Outcaste, "bhangra" is defined in this way: "the Punjabi dance form that mutated from farming and work songs into the dominant genre of Asian pop played at everything from weddings to nightclubs."[21] It is out of this Punjabi tradition that Apache Indian's rajamuffin *stylee* mutates.

In "Chok There," the blistering first cut on his debut CD *No Reservations,* Apache Indian assumes the hybrid persona of "Don Raja," a Don Gorgon Indian rajamuffin who "bring[s] a new stylee" and a "different fashion." It is hyperbolic self-aggrandizement on a grand scale. Apache Indian, appropriating all of the rhetorical conventions of Jamaican ragamuffin DJ discourse, deploys them to voice his particular cultural location at the dangerous crossroads:

> No. 1 in a the Bombay chart,
> Indian me a tear them apart,
> When me come me bring a new stylee,
> So listen crowd a people and you have to follow me
> Chok There,
> Them a ball[22] when they see the Indian
> Chok There,
> Ragamuffin under style and pattern,
> Chok There
> When me come that a different fashion
> First tune me a say me do it reach No. 1
> In a the reggae charts and the Indian
> Chok There
> See me face apon the television
> Chok There
> Hear me voice pon the radio station
> Promoter them a come them a rub off them hand
> Keeping a session and them want it fi ram
> Put me name pon the invitation
> Pon the gate go raise a million
> Me bring a brand new style apon the island

Fe the black a fe white and a fe the Indian

So each and every one come follow fashion

Dip you knee cork[23] out you bottom

Everyone in a the Bhangra fashion.[24]

In "Come Follow Me," Apache Indian, sensitive to his multiethnic audience—"fe the black a fe white and a fe the Indian"—declares that "[him] come fi mix di Indian, man, with the Patwa."[25] This lexical mix becomes an obvious metaphor for a process of acculturation that is the by-product of the immigrant experience in Britain. It is also a by-product of African/Indian acculturation in the Caribbean and South America. Writing about the processes of language adaptation in Guyana, the linguist John Rickford asks a pertinent question:

> How did the Indians' acculturation to the Creole language and culture take place? It is commonly asserted that the Indian gradually acquired the Creole English of the Africans with whom they worked on the sugar estates.*. . . One factor that must have been important in the linguistic assimilation of the Indian immigrants, as it was for the African immigrants of the same period, was the emergence of Indian creoles, children born in the colony and acquiring the Creole English around them as a first language.[26]

In a footnote at the asterisk Rickford inserts,

> Bronkhurst (1881:15) notes that "the newly imported coolies find it difficult for a time to make themselves understood, but they manage it somehow or other when they converse with black creole labourers on the different estates." He also observes (p. 53) that "all [the Indian immigrants] learn the creole patois or corrupted English, and seem fonder of talking it than their own beautiful and poetic language, the Tamil. In visiting, I have come upon some Indian families where the children could not speak their native languages, but only creole."

The parallel "creolization" processes in the Caribbean and the United Kingdom problematize conventional regional (mis)conceptions of "creolization" as a peculiarly "New World" phenomenon. In Apache Indian's Birmingham, that multicultural city of immigrants, the "creolization" process, more familiarly studied in the context of the colonies of Britain, assumes new dynamics in the very belly of the beast of empire. Nevertheless, "creolization" is, at its core, nothing more or less than the inevitable cultural adaptations that result from culture contact.

In "Don Raja," the final cut on his first CD, Apache Indian positions himself as interpreter between mutually unintelligible discourses:

> Them a talk bout Donness and Don Dada and
> Donnette are you sister or mother
> Them a talk bout Don Gorgon
> Come fe rule the area
> But where me come from them can't understand
> Them kind of lingwar
> So me have fe take a bran new style over India
> Me are the Don, Me are the [*sic*][27]

As translator, Apache Indian not only explains Jamaican/Black British culture to Indians; he also explains Indian culture to outsiders. He thus opens up a space for mutual understanding, foregrounding the role of the emotive language of music in facilitating communication, however superficial, in contexts where verbal meaning is often elusive.

In "Come Follow Me" the DJ assumes the role of tour guide to India, responding to DJ Mr. Mikey G's challenge to demonstrate his knowledge of "his" country. Admittedly, Apache Indian initially paints a rather touristy picture of India:

> See the Taj Mahal one of the seven wonder
> The golden temple a Amritsar

But you can't reach the-so till you cross the water

The Hindus bath[e] in-a the Ganges river

In-a Bombay city you find the film star

The nicest place are [a] the one Kashmir

Himalaya mountain by the Chinese border[28]

Apache Indian does move from the wonderful perspective of the wide-eyed tourist to touch briefly on political and economic issues:

Say the seek [Sikh] them a fight fe Kalistania

In-a Pindand city nough people suffer

The greeb them a beg fe food and water

And if you pass one place where them call Calcutta

Be sure to leave a dollar fe the snake Charma

So you take it from the youth the originator

Me are the first Dj from out of India

So each and every one come listen and follow[29]

In an interview with Jerry Pinto, given during his 1993 tour of India to promote *No Reservations,* Apache Indian discloses his sense of alienation on the borderline between hostile camps:

There was even a problem when I was singing. The Indian community felt that I was being disrespectful to the culture and a traitor to the community and to the country as a whole because of what I was doing and the manner in which I was singing it—reggae. They relate that to the black sub-culture which they see as violent and drug-related. But when they saw that I was proud to be an Indian, that I was not being disrespectful but just talking about important issues, that was settled. The black community felt I was using reggae to make a lot of money. But then when they listened to the music, when they listened to the interviews, when they saw that I had a genuine love of reggae, that settled down.[30]

In his transgressive border crossings, Apache Indian playfully/cunningly misrepresents himself as a composite American/Arawak/Apache Indian. In "Make Way for the Indian," the DJ, in combination with African American rapper Tim Dog, declares his mastery of disguise:

Tim Dog:

I say one two three

Make way for the Indian

Lick shots for the Rajah

Apache:

Dis a one rude raggamuffin Indian

Wid di mike inna mi hand a man a look how mi tan

[I'm holding the mike, and people recognise my power]

Dis a one rude raggamuffin Indian

Wid di mike inna mi hand mi come fi nice di nation

Mi a di Indian rest in mi wigwam

No time fi romp, man,

Wid dem deh tin pan

Paint pon mi face, man

Drum dem fi beat pan

Feather mi head band

. . .

Smoke signal a dem fly inna di sky

Indian fi now, a next cowboy fi die

My time fi shot a boy, a your time fi cry[31]

Jerry Pinto asks Apache Indian a provocative series of questions about this racial/ethnic cross-dressing:

Why Apache? (We have to keep this quick.)

The name comes from the Wild Apache Supercut [*sic*]. I used to listen to him a lot and he's a good friend now.

But that makes you a confluence of three cultures: the British, the Indian and the Red Indian. Isn't that a bit polyglot even for you?

Yeah, that was a bit of a problem in the beginning specially when the album No Reservations came out because the Red Indians were fighting for no reservations at the time. But that was good in a kind of a way because it helped the album. They identified with it in a way.

But it might seem that you were seeking to be identified with a country other than your own, in a way, hiding your real ethnic origin with a little fancy naming.

I don't think that's true. I've always been proud to be an Indian and I've always said so.[32]

In "Badd Indian" Apache Indian boasts in a bombastic style that fuses the Jamaican dancehall mode of verbal badness with yet another Caribbean vernacular tradition, Trinidadian "robber talk." Donning the mask of Native American Indian—a recurring masquerade figure in the Trinidad carnival—Apache Indian assumes several layers of subterfuge:

Bad B Bad Bad Bad Indian and if a bwoy
Try a thing them there have fe drop
With me bow and arrow hitch up there pon me back
Say me arrow to me bow then me pull the arrow back
And when me let it go cowboy them a drop.
Me say take it from Apache Indian when me chat
From the top a where me start from the bottom where me stop
When me go a Canada me a launch and [sic] attack
Capture the arawak put me in a cell block
Me no mind how them talk, me no mind how them chat
If a bwoy try a thing them there youth have fe drop
Say the sheriff him a come mon with a ranger

9 and 16 cock to fire

But you take Apache bare back rider

Round the back a fe me head a no me have two feather[33]

Apache Indian's reference to his tour of Canada foregrounds the circulation of dancehall culture in the Caribbean diaspora in North America. There yet another Apache, this one born in Guyana—"Apache Waria"—asserts the potency of yet another adaptation of rajamuffin discourse, now mixed with a soca beat. In the undated CD, *The Best of Apache Waria,* the DJ assumes the standard guises of his Jamaican mentors. "Agony"—male sexual prowess—is celebrated. For example, on the track "Mention," performed with "Arawak," Apache Waria asserts:

Oh God, man, Apache an Arawak Indian come

Full up a style an full up a pattern

Mr Mention fi di area don [?]

Through shi want di loving a pon di Guyanese don

Di Indian inna di Caribbean

Inna shi punaani, don, shi want di Indian

Everywhe mi go di Indian a mention

Shi want di Arawak fi live inna her mansion

Cau shi want di buddy from di Indian man

Shi no want Shabba Ranks.[34]

Sexual rivalry between African and Indian men, a recurring feature of sexual politics in Trinidad and Guyana, is playfully resolved to the advantage of the Indian in this song. Hyperbole is a characteristic feature of the DJ's repertoire both in the indigenous Jamaican context and its appropriations elsewhere. In addition, food metaphors recur in dancehall lyrics; the appetite for food and sex seems insatiable. So Apache Waria celebrates Guyanese women in vivid curry tones:

> All a di Guyanese girls dem
> Mi love unu like cook food
> Just like di curry goat an di dahlpouri.

The generic Jamaican metaphor of "cook food" becomes elaborated as the culturally specific East Indian cuisine of Apache Waria's desire.

On his third CD, *Real People,* Apache Indian continues to demonstrate full control over the dancehall idiom. The lyrics of "Jump Up" invite the audience to participate in the eruption of the celebratory dance; the song simultaneously proclaims Apache Indian's authority as the don:

> Don Indian me come fe mash up again
> Lyrics a fire and that me defend
> All the bad mind them have fe back off me friend
> A now me come set de new trend
> Send them all a message fe warn them again
> Test the Rajah yu ina problem
> Push we culture a that me intend
> Run the circuit once again SLAM!
>
> . . .
>
> You wan test the Don make sure you ready
> Indian deh back with the authority
> Set the order ina community
> This is the way fe do it BOMB![35]

Apache's reference to "order ina community" not only signals his authoritative position as number one in the ranking order of performers. It also alludes to the DJ's recognition of the need for the community to be restored to order as it fights against destructive social forces. So in "Mention" the DJ chants down the drug-pushing, gun-toting gangsters who have no respect for any authority whatsoever:

Chorus:

Listen ca me come fe mention

All the badness that need correction

All the youth them that need direction

The innocent suffer and need protection (repeat)

Verse 1:

Beca the youth them 'pon the street them have no manner[s]

Them no respect themselves or a fe them elder

Wan walk 'pon the street like them a gangster

And a carry fe them tool like them a soldier

But check it me bredrin it out a order

Say how them could a thief from the old grandmother

Them lef her fe dead fe just two dollar

The weak and defenseless ina fe we area

The boy them are so coward no the boy them are so slack

Mash up the place when we just build it back

The innocent people dem wan fe attack

All the badness it fe stop.[36]

Apache Indian's concern for the restoration of civil society extends beyond the immediate streets of Britain's cities. The DJ invites members of the Indian diaspora to turn their attention "back home" to the continent. In "India (A.I.F.)" [Apache Indian Foundation] the DJ asks an unsettling question:

> Well do you really know what's going on ina India?
> And do you really know what's going on back home?
> Well do you really know what's going on in your country?
> What we did lose let me tell you it's that has to get found.[37]

The liner notes inform us that: "This song has been especially written for the Apache Indian Foundation (A.I.F.) which is a fully registered charity organisation based in Mumbai, India. The foundation has been set up to provide relief for under-privileged and disabled children, financial assistance to schools, colleges, libraries, orphanages and other institutions that help children in India."

The first verse of the song details the suffering and appeals to the "crowd of people," the conventional dancehall designation for the audience, to listen and respond appropriately:

> Like ina Mumbai and in Calcutta
> We have [fe] think bout all them that suffer
> And down in the ghetto dem cross India
> Sing out me friend and say a prayer
> Every morning them a get up them a starve and suffer
> Have fe hussle and a juggle right pon the corner
> Have fe beg a rupee fe little bread and water
> Have fe look and search fe find a shelter
> So listen crowd of people ca me done have me plan
> In a India set the foundation
> Fe help all the poor, needy an orphan
> Fe help all the charity that support the young
> So everybody cross the world have fe come together
> Have fe think bout the youth that need fe prosper
> Have fe lend a little hand fe build the future
> Worldwide support fe Mother India.[38]

"Mother India," like "the old grandmother" in "Mention," must be protected from predators.

In a nice juxtapositioning, "Raag Ragga," the next cut on the *Real People* CD, revises the image of India as charity case. Instead, it is the musical heritage of the continent that is celebrated. The somewhat inaccurate liner notes underscore the eclecticism of the musical mix: "This track combines Apache's unique style of Ragga with the use of four styles of Indian Classical singing in the form of specific scales, each known as a Raag. The Raags sung by Vishwa Prakash Ji, accompanied by Sashi Chopra, first commence with the 'Dhrupad' style which then emerges into the second raag, known as 'Khyaal.' The third raag presented is 'Mishra,' which matches the melody of the song and then leads on to the 'Karnatak' style, which is South Indian singing, delivered in half and quarter notes."

The Raag/Ragga near pun is a fitting metaphor for the cross-cultural fusion music that Apache Indian creates. He mixes the Indian with the patwa and appeals to a global audience. Somewhat ironically, the Jamaican posse is not named in the roll call:

> Me come fe Big Up the posse them ina India
>
> In a Mumbai and in Calcutta
>
> Down a Madras and in a Agra
>
> In Bangalore and a Amritsar
>
> Big Up the crew them in America
>
> In a Japan and cross Africa
>
> In a England and in Canada
>
> Shout again fe the Don Rajah.[39]

But perhaps Apache Indian does not need to name his Jamaican antecedents, as he speaks with their tongue. In the interview with Pinto, the DJ acknowledges the inevitability of his instinctual choice of the Jamaican language, seasoned with Punjabi, for his performance of the identity of DJ:

> **About the language that you use. Do you see it as an appropriation of the English language? The creation of a new dialect?**
>
> No. I sing as it comes to me. I can't sing it any other way.
>
> **So you don't think you'd ever be able to sing a straight English song?**

No.

Why not?

Because even if I did sing one and it did become a hit, I'd find it very difficult to keep up. I get behind the mike and I sing. And I sing in this patois.

So a pure Punjabi song in reggae would also be out?

No. It doesn't work that way. Seeing the response in India, I've composed a song with only Punjabi words and I'll sing it while I'm here.[40]

The title of Apache Indian's fourth CD, *Karma,* seems to signify the DJ's acceptance of his fate as a man destined to crisscross contested borders and engage in sound clashes. The opening duet with Boy George, who so flamboyantly resists conventional definitions of masculinity, proclaims Apache Indian's freedom to establish musical alliances as he sees fit:

Apache Indian:
Ghetto man talk, weh di ghetto man sing
Cau you know seh down inna di ghetto
Weh di youth dem need di blessing, man
All Indian massive unu hold tight!

Boy George:
In a cold and gray Chicago morn
A poor little baby child is born
In the ghetto

Apache Indian:
Right down inna di ghetto
Weh di youth dem a cry
Mek wi tell dem now ya rude boy

Boy George:
In the ghetto

Apache Indian:

Tell dem fi me no Mr G!

Leggo di riddim ya man[41]

Apache Indian's critique of the depraved conditions in which ghetto youth eke out an existence explicitly acknowledges the entrenched culture of violence, exacerbated by easy access to debilitating, illegal drugs:

Live inna di ghetto it no fun

Di youth dem ha fi carry fi dem knife an gun

Di drugs dem a push but wi no waan none

Ha fi clean up di ghetto fi wi daughter an son

Why?

Mi no waan see di youth cry

Like inna Calcutta an down a Mumbai

Cau all dem a struggle an a try dem a try

But wha dem a go do a when di well run dry?[42]

There are no easy answers to the pervasive dilemmas of ghetto youth. For example, Apache Indian makes it clear in "Religion" that he disdains organized religion and the terrors perpetuated in the name of religiosity. Distinguishing between "respect" and fanaticism, the DJ somewhat ambiguously confesses: "I & I respect all religion/ But mi seh mi can't follow one."[43] Single-minded religious affiliation is likely to lead to "war and contradiction." In "Calling out to Jah," his duet with the singer Luciano, Apache Indian declares his valorization of the "peace an love" philosophy of Rastafari, thus crossing yet another ideological border. Apache Indian echoes Luciano's evocation of Marcus Garvey's philosophy: "One God, one aim, one destiny": "Seh one God mi have, one destination/ Respect each other and love can reign."

In sing-jay style, Luciano delineates the philosophy of unity and Apache responds affirmatively:

Luciano:

In this world of uncertainty

All we've got is a you and me

Apache Indian:

A just you an me yu know brethren

Luciano:

There's no need for hostility

Let's unite to live in love and Inity

Say brothers and sisters

Apache:

I say brothers and sisters

Luciano:

No matter what denomination

No matter the class or the creed

Apache:

All nation

Luciano:

And no matter your nation

Apache:

That's right

Luciano:

Is one God, one aim, one destiny

One universal, can't you see?

Apache:

Oh can't you see?

Luciano:

Come along let's unite

Apache:
Let's unite

Luciano:
Let's unite to live in love and Inity

Apache:
Right

Luciano:
Dat's why we

Luciano & Apache:
Calling out to Jah

Apache:
Calling out to di highest father

Luciano & Apache:
Wi calling out to Jah

Luciano:
Apache mi bredrin come sing!

In response to Luciano's cue, Apache Indian elaborates in Jamaican Luciano's message that had been sung in English. In this *upful* duet, the dancehall convention of the singer using English and the DJ chanting in Jamaican somewhat ironically underscores Apache Indian's smooth passage across linguistic barriers: The Jamaican singer is the one who uses English and the English DJ performs in Jamaican.

Whether African or whether Indian
Remember Rastafari seh di whole wi a one
Seh whether you be black or white or whether yu be brown
Seh I & I come ya so fi mek you settle down
Wid di love inna mi heart an di voice from mi thought

Wid di words from mi mouth, hear di Rastafari shout
An mi seh peace an love, come mek we spread it about
Me no want no inner war from east west down to south
Weh mi seh?
East and West unu better come together, gether
Member seh di whole a we a brether, brether, brether
Easy, Luciano from yu a di messenger
Di two a we together ha fi set di order.[44]

Trinidadian novelist Earl Lovelace envisages an optimistic model of African/Indian acculturation such as is accomplished in the emergence of rajamuffin discourse in Britain. It is Lovelace's Pariag who muses about the possibility of orchestrating a new music with both the instruments brought across the Atlantic and those produced on the further shores of Africa and India in the Caribbean:

. . . I wish I did walk with a flute or a sitar, and walk in right there in the middle of the steelband yard where they was making new drums, new sounds, a new music from rubbish tins and bits of steel and oil drums, bending the iron over fire, chiselling out new notes. New notes. I wish I woulda go in there where they was making their life anew in fire, with chisel and hammer, and sit down with my sitar on my knee and say: Fellars, this is me, Pariag from New Lands. Gimme the key! Give me the Do Re Mi. Run over the scale. Leh We Fa Sol La! Gimme the beat, lemme beat! Listen to these strings.[45]

In the words of Pariag, Lovelace acknowledges the fact that cultural accommodation does not require dissolution of cultural identity:

And he smiled, thinking of Miss Cleothilda and her All o' we is one. No. We didn't have to melt into one. I woulda be me for my own self. A beginning.

A self to go in the world with, with something in my hands to give. We wouldn't have to melt into one. They woulda see me.[46]

Steve Kapur, the former welder from Handsworth, is still bending the iron over fire. Not waiting to be given the key or the beat, he has had the courage to do what Pariag only dreamed of. He boldly inserts himself into the discourse of Jamaican migrants in Handsworth, Birmingham. Making a space for himself and others, claiming visibility, Apache Indian creates a hybrid sound that voices the polyphonic reality of those living in/between. Somewhat paradoxically, he celebrates his accomplishment in the contradictory language of both militant gun salute and domesticated culinary allusion. These seemingly dissonant metaphors articulate the DJ's eclectic sensibility, fed on both native and imported fare:

> Well here wi come again
> Fi lick a shot fi di Indian ragamuffin posse
> An Ah want yu know say
> Apache Indian is hotter than the vindaloo curry[47]

The Dancehall Transnation

Language, Lit/orature, and Global Jamaica

(co-author Hubert Devonish)

The norm that is accepted in the international community is that a state should ideally be made up of a single national/ethnic group speaking a single language. Such notions have their origins in the Europe of the late Middle Ages, following the breakup of the Holy Roman Empire. This ideal of what a state should be has spread across the world in the wake of European expansion and domination and has been universally accepted in spite of the fact that the states that appeared in Europe hardly ever fit the model. For a state to survive, those over whom control is exercised generally have to accept the legitimacy of that state. Its citizens, therefore, have to be presented with a body of ideological justifications for the existence of the state and its authority. One such justification is that the state is the highest expression of a shared national identitiy.

The claim that this identity exists is based on cultural characteristics that are considered to be common to members of the group but not to others. Where a common national identity does not exist, it is usually suggested that such an identity is in the process of being forged. Another justification is that within the state there exists a common language that permits communication between all citizens of the state. Where such a common language manifestly does not exist, the governing groups propose that it is emerging and/or being spread as part of the process of nation building. National identity and language identity become linked when, as often happens, one of the cultural features a national group claims to share is a common language.

The notion of "a language" is itself a cultural construct. Speakers of a series of related language varieties may, at a particular point in their history, come to view these speech forms as belonging to a single entity, a language. These speakers begin to perceive this shared language both as a medium of communication among themselves and as a means of distinguishing members of their own group from members of other groups. Several factors may trigger the change in language consciousness that gives rise to the notion that a language exists. One such factor is the appearance of *written* language.

Purely oral languages do have some disadvantages. Up until the twentieth century, speakers of nonwritten languages could not communicate with each other unless they were within earshot. Writing is a form of technology for representing language that circumvents this difficulty. The reader does not need to be present at the time and place where the writer produced the message. A written language message has as a potential audience anyone who can gain access to the surface on which the written symbols have been marked. In reality, of course, such access is restricted. Only two options exist. One could physically transport oneself to the place where the written message is located. Otherwise, potential readers could have the written language message physically transported to them.

Printing solved the dilemma of restricted access to single written bodies of language messages. It created the possibility of multiple copies of the same language message. Access was not now limited to the original form of the message. The existence of multiple copies increased several times over the size of the potential audience for any written message. With all its obvious advantages, writing, particularly when enhanced by the application of printing technology, came to be perceived by speakers as the primary form of language. It was a short step from this perception to the conclusion that only those forms of speech that can and do appear in writing and print are true languages.

In societies possessing writing, nearly all use of the prestige language in public formal situations has its origins in writing. Public speeches, lectures, and news broadcasts, for example, are produced mainly by speakers reading scripts aloud to an audience. In diglossic situations, language consciousness becomes focused around the "high" language used in public, formal, written, and literary contexts. Indeed, the primary function of diglossia for that section of the population that controls the "high" language is to preserve a monopoly over both the prestige language and writing itself.

"Low" language varieties, spoken in private and informal situations, have no recognition as constituting a language in and of themselves. The reasoning that gives rise to this perception is that such varieties have no writing system and, therefore, no literature. Consequently, they do not constitute a language. At best, when recognized as being different from the "high" language, they are regarded as broken forms of that language or of some other language that possesses writing and literature. Literature is produced when language is used creatively in the written medium.

Purely oral forms of verbal creativity—for example proverb, folk tale, and popular song—that have their origins in the language of the "low" culture tend to be devalued in the conservative, monopolist discourse of literates. The combination of creativity and written language produces strong feelings of emotional identification in many speech communities. Literature creates a focus for the language consciousness of members of the speech community. It provides them with an ideal image of what the language is or ought to be.

In Jamaica, diglossia is a long-established feature of the language situation. A cluster of language varieties occupy the position of "high" language in the diglossia. These are varieties that members of the speech community identify as English. In popular consciousness, these varieties have the characteristic that they are "a language." English has all of the features that a language is supposed to possess. Among these is a standard and well-known writing system and a solid body of global literature. The English literary tradition dates back to Chaucer, Shakespeare, Milton, and the King James Version of the Bible.

The position as the "low" language in the diglossia is occupied by language varieties that members of the speech community would describe as "patwa," "dialect," "bad English," and "broken English." These are varieties that linguists often grace with the term "Jamaican Creole." For political reasons, we use this term interchangeably with "Jamaican." These "nonstandard" varieties traditionally do not appear in the writing of native speakers. They consequently have no literature.

Jamaican linguists Jean D'Costa and Barbara Lalla confirm that as early as 1740, "connected discourses" in Jamaican appeared in print.[1] The early recorders of Jamaican were, most often, expatriate British writers who were fascinated with native life and wished to document its curiosities as accurately as possible. One such curiosity was African-derived polygamy. Robert Charles Dallas's *The History of the Maroons* (1803) records a conversation between a Jamaican Maroon and a proselytizing Christian, attempting to convert the Maroon from polygamy:

> "Top, Massa Governor," said he, "top lilly bit—you say me mus forsake my wife."—"Only one of them."—"Which dat one? Jesus Christ say so? Gar a'mighty say so? No, no, massa; Gar a'mighty good; he no tell somebody he mus forsake him wife and children. Somebody no wicked for forsake him wife! No, massa, dis here talk no do for we."[2]

Dallas, recognizing Jamaican as a distinct language, offers an English translation:

In other language thus: "Stay, Sir," said the Maroon, "stay a little. You tell me that I must forsake my wife."—"Only one of them."—"And which shall that be? Does Jesus Christ say so? Does God say so? No, no Sir; God is good, and allows no one to forsake his wife and children. He who forsakes his wife must be a wicked man. This is a doctrine, Sir, not suited to us."[3]

Given the intention in all these cases to record and document actual speech that had been heard, there is some question as to whether most of these could qualify as literature—creative written language in Jamaican Creole.

There does exist in these Jamaican Creole language varieties, however, an established body of creative *oral* language. But Jamaica is a society that requires that varieties possess writing before they gain a place in public consciousness as constituting a language. Jamaican Creole varieties, therefore, fail the language test. They cannot be recognized as constituting a language in their own right. The most liberal traditional position assigned to them, as a result of the similarity in their vocabulary with English, is that of a dialect of English. The English language proper is perceived as being made up of those varieties that have writing and an established literature.

In Jamaica, there is a long tradition of creative writing in European languages, mostly in English and some Latin. The extraordinary Franciscus Williams is the eighteenth-century precursor of succeeding generations of literate Jamaicans who defined their humanity in terms of their ability to master "learned speech."[4] Williams, to whom Edward Long devotes a chapter in his multivolume *History of Jamaica,* is a classic example of this early type. According to Long, Williams, ". . . being a boy of unusual lively parts, was pitched upon to be the subject of an experiment, which it is said, the Duke of Montagu was curious to make, in order to discover, whether by proper cultivation, and a regular course of tuition at school and the university, a Negroe might be found as capable of literature as a white person."[5]

In his Latin "Ode" to George Haldane, Esq., short-lived governor of Jamaica (the English translation is Edward Long's), Williams anticipates the preoccupations of later elitist-nationalist Jamaican poets writing in European languages. He may live in the tropics, not England, and his body, like that of his Black Muse, may be "clad in sable vest," but he is nevertheless culturally "white" because of his eloquent control of European language and literature. Linking color, race, national identity, language, and letters, Williams assimilates into western culture. He thus proves himself worthy of self-government in pre-emancipation Jamaica:

We live, alas! where the bright god of day,

Full from the zenith whirls his torrid ray:

Beneath the rage of his consuming fires,

All fancy melts, all eloquence expires.

Yet may you deign accept this humble song,

Tho' wrapt in gloom, and from a falt'ring tongue;

Tho' dark the stream on which the tribute flows,

Not from the skin, but from the heart it rose.

To all of human kind benignant heaven

(Since nought forbids) one common soul has given.

This rule was 'stablish'd by th'Eternal Mind;

Nor virtue's self, nor prudence are confin'd

To colour; none imbues the honest heart;

To science none belongs, and none to art.

Oh! Muse, of blackest tint, why shrinks thy breast,

Why fears t'approach the Caesar of the West!

Dispel thy doubts, with confidence ascend

The regal dome, and hail him for thy friend:

Nor blush, altho' in garb funereal drest,

Thy body's white, tho' clad in sable vest.

Manners unsullied, and the radiant glow

Of genius, burning with desire to know;

And learned speech, with modest accent worn,

Shall best the sooty African adorn.

An heart with wisdom fraught, a patriot flame,

A love of virtue; these shall lift his name

Conspicuous far, beyond his kindred race,

Distinguished from them by the foremost place.[6]

In this context, the work of the prolific early-twentieth-century novelist Herbert DeLisser must be noted, particularly since he authored *Jane's Career*, the first Jamaican novel in which the central character is a native speaker of Jamaican Creole. That novel, published in 1914, marked another stage in the representation of Jamaican Creole in written texts. Bilingual native Jamaicans were beginning to represent in their own written texts the reported speech of native speakers of Jamaican. Somewhat like the early non-native recorders of eighteenth- and nineteenth-century Jamaican Creole speech, DeLisser faithfully documented Jane's speech as a kind of curiosity—local color.

By the 1930s, there was an intensification of effort in Jamaica to contribute to the body of literature already existing in English. The material was inspired by life in Jamaica and the Caribbean and language varieties in use in the country. Most of this material, which was in those varieties identified as English by the community, came from the small minority who, like the eighteenth-century Franciscus Williams, had both literary skills and a high level of competence in these English varieties. The *Focus* literary magazine, published in 1943, 1948, 1956, and 1960 and first edited by Edna Manley, the English sculptor and painter who was married to Norman Washington Manley, founder of the People's National Party, reflected an insurgent Jamaican nationalism.

This literary production was the result of significant changes in the consciousness of the Jamaican educated elite. They were beginning to see themselves as having a national identity and a set of regional interests distinct from those of the ruling British colonial elite. As an expression of this consciousness, they were producing literature in local varieties of English—language varieties they themselves used and with which they were identified. There was another aspect of this literary production: The vast majority of the population were speakers of varieties of Jamaican Creole who had little or no command of English. The literature produced, therefore, also served to mark off the educated elite from the majority of the Jamaican population.

The literary output in local varieties of English thus marked the emergence of a sense of national identity centered around the educated elite. The monolingual Creole-speaking population was peripheral to this consciousness. According to elite perception, the mass of the population would have to be brought out of the dark into the light. With enlightened government, they would be taught literacy and acquire competence in English. The educated elite, aided by this new sense of national identity, was able to lead a movement that culminated in the achievement of self-government and, eventually, political independence. The state thus created was based on a sense of national identity shared by a marginal elite—to the exclusion of the vast majority of the population.

There were some limited efforts on the part of those who were literate in English to produce literature exclusively in the varieties of Jamaican Creole. The first such documented efforts were those of Claude McKay who was encouraged to experiment by Walter Jekyll, an English aristocrat and intellectual resident in Jamaica. McKay recalls Jekyll's enthusiastic response to one of his early poems written in Jamaican:

All those poems that I gave him to read had been done in straight English, but there was one short one about an ass that was laden for the market— laden with native vegetables—who had suddenly sat down in the middle of the road and wouldn't get up. Its owner was talking to it in the Jamaican dialect, telling it to get up. That was the poem that Mr. Jekyll was laughing about. He then told me that he did not like my poems in straight English— they were repetitious. "But this," said he, holding up the donkey poem, "this is the real thing. The Jamaican dialect has never been put into literary form except in my Annancy stories. Now is your chance as a native boy [to] put the Jamaica dialect into literary language. I am sure your poems will sell."[7]

Not surprisingly, McKay was mystified by Jekyll's response: "I was not very enthusiastic about this statement, because to us who were getting education in the English schools the Jamaican dialect was considered a vulgar tongue. It was the language of the peasants. All cultivated people spoke English, straight English."[8] Nevertheless, he went on to write two collections of "dialect poetry" that proved to be very influential.[9] Louise Bennett, who followed in his footsteps, recorded in print traditional Jamaican Creole Anansi stories. In addition, she produced a large body of original writing, mainly poetry/dramatic monologues, in the language. She acknowledges McKay as a role model, as noted in the following account: "It was during this period of high unemployment, labour unrest and Garveyism that Louise first saw Jamaican creole language in print. When she was about seven years old, a teacher at Calabar School in Kingston (Miss Dukes), knowing the child was always telling her classmates Anancy stories, gave her a copy of Claude McKay's *Constab Ballads* (1912), saying, 'Here are some verses a man wrote in the Jamaican talk. You must read some of them. They're very funny!'"[10]

Several of Louise Bennett's poems satirize the elitist nationalist movement for independence. For example, "Independance" (the pun on dance derides the "song and dance" of the occasion) wittily contrasts the ordinary Jamaican's sense of self-importance with the government's newly acquired status as independent nation. Bennett emphasizes the disparity between official conceptions of the nation-state and the everyday, small-scale politics of individual empowerment:

Independance is we nature
Born an bred in all we do,

An she glad fe se[e] dat Govament

Tun independant to [*sic*].[11]

There were two difficulties facing Bennett in her attempts to write in Jamaican. Her readership was made up of literates like herself. Anyone who had acquired literacy had done so in English. There was no perception within any sector of the population that a linguistic system other than English existed in Jamaica. For example, Professor the Honorable Rex Nettleford, in his 1966 introduction to Bennett's *Jamaica Labrish,* describes her experimental creative writing in Jamaican Creole thus—with a measure of irony one supposes: "In a quarter of a century she has carved designs out of the shapeless and unruly substance that is the Jamaican dialect."[12] Nettleford, as a schoolboy at Cornwall College, himself carved dialect verse in the style of Louise Bennett. The metaphor of the plastic arts further alienates Jamaican Creole from conventional discourses of what constitutes a language. Unlike real languages, which have shape and rules (and grammar), and which do not behave in an unseemly fashion, Jamaican Creole is a promiscuous "idiom whose limitations as a bastard tongue are all too evident."[13]

Bennett's struggle, in the first instance, was to achieve "dialect" status for this shapeless and unruly bastard tongue, as is expressed in her satirical poem "Bans o' Killing":

Jamaican:

Ef yuh dah-equal up wid English

Language, den wha meck

Yu gwine go feel inferior, wen

It come to dialect?

If yuh kean sing "Linstead Market"

An "Wata come a me y'eye",

Yuh wi haffi tap sing "Auld lang syne"

An "Comin thru de rye".
Dah language weh yuh proud o',
Weh yu honour and respeck,
Po' Mass Charlie! Yuh no know sey
Dat it spring from dialect! [14]

English:
If you want to measure up to English
Then just tell me
Why are you going to feel inferior,
When it comes to this business of dialect?

If you can't sing "Linstead Market"
And "Water come a me y'eye",
You'll have to stop singing "Auld lang syne"
And "Coming through the rye".

That language which you're so proud of,
Which you honour and respect,
Poor Mr. Charlie! Don't you know
That it sprang from a dialect! [15]

Her persuasive argument was that English-speaking communities in Britain had regional dialects. The fact that Jamaica also had a regional dialect should be acknowledged without embarrassment.

Given her ideas at the time about language, Bennett adopted the conventions of English nonstandard dialect writing, replete with apostrophes and alterations to normal spelling not justified by any pronunciation difference. She thus employed the notoriously inconsistent conventions of the English writing system to represent a language that had a sound system quite distinct from that of English. Her decision to write Jamaican and her choice of writing system achieved her immediate objective of giving

Jamaican Creole "dialect" status amongst the literate English-speaking elite.

Later, moving beyond the limiting conception of Jamaican as a bastard dialect of English, Louise Bennett herself contested the popular "corruption of language" view of Jamaican. In "Jamaica Language," which she performs on her album *Yes M'Dear—Miss Lou Live*, Bennett argues humorously that English is just as "corrupt" as Jamaican since it is derived in part from Norman French, Greek, and Latin.[16] Jamaican should be recognized as similarly "derived" from other languages: "English is a derivation but Jamaica dialec is corruption! What a unfairity."[17] Further, Bennett now gives a more complicated genealogy for "Jamaica dialec" that extends the origins of the language beyond the dialect-of-English genesis. The African linguistic heritage is acknowledged and its subversive ethos is celebrated.

The emergence of Jamaican Creole is now conceived as the end result of a radical political process. The new language is a cunning, revolutionary assertion of African verbal creativity and cultural autonomy. But Bennnett's inclusion of "we English forefahders" in the Creole family history craftily acknowledges the English elements in Jamaican Creole and simultaneously underscores the "mus-an-boun" deculturating compulsion that is an essential element of the enslavement process. Bennett also derides the limitations of the English colonizers who could not master the African languages:

> For Jamaican Dialec did start when we English forefahders did start mus-an-boun we African ancestors fi stop talk fi-dem African Language altogedder an learn fi talk so-so English, because we English forefahders couldn understan what we African ancestors-dem wasa seh to dem one anodder when dem wasa talk eena dem African Language to dem one annodder!
>
> But we African ancestors-dem pop we English forefahders-dem. Yes! Pop dem an disguise up de English Language fi projec fi-dem African Language in such a way dat we English forefahders-dem still couldn

understan what we African ancestors-dem wasa talk bout when dem wasa
talk to dem one annodder![18]

Having tested the limitations of the corrupt bastard language,
Jamaican, Bennett has succeeded in helping to legitimize it. Part of the
legitimizing process has been the writing down of the language. Bennett
herself insists that she is a writer: "From the beginning, nobody ever
recognised me as a writer. 'Well, she is 'doing' dialect'; it wasn't even
writing you know. Up to now a lot of people don't even think I write."[19]
But the choice of an inappropriate writing system had an important
additional effect. Many persons who were literate in English and also
spoke Jamaican Creole could claim with some justification that Jamaican
Creole material was difficult to read. Such claims emphasized the
superiority of the standard "language," English, relative to its nonstandard "dialect," Jamaican Creole.

The production of Jamaican Creole material in an English writing
system had another difficulty. The only people who could read it were, of
course, the literates. However, all of these had acquired their reading and
writing skills in English. Thus, even the Creole material that Bennett was
writing was ending up with largely the same readership as that written in
Jamaican varieties of English. The work by Bennett and similar other
writers could not initially, therefore, become the focal point of a language
consciousness among the majority of the population who were nonliterate
speakers of Jamaican.

The strategy deployed by Bennett to circumvent this problem was
public performance of her work. From the point of view of trying to create
a Jamaican Creole language consciousness, however, there was enormous
difficulty. The very fact that this material was reaching a mass audience in
an oral form and not in writing only served to confirm existing popular
attitudes. Even illiterates shared the view that the special category of "a
language" was reserved for language varieties that could be shown to be
widely written.

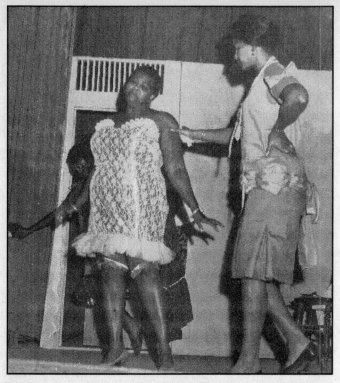

Down to the basics: In this scene from the Little Theatre Movement's 1963 panto-
mime, "Queenie's Daughter," the Society dressmaker (Lois Kelly-Barrow), gives
instructions to Miss Queenie (Louise Bennett) on the proper posture for upward
social mobility. Miss Bennett's costume anticipates dancehall aesthetics and the scene
evokes the transformation of Marcia in the 1997 film *Dancehall Queen*. Photo:
Gleaner Archives, 1963.

An important potential solution to the writing system dilemma
became available in 1961 with the publication of *Jamaica Talk* by the
linguist Frederic Cassidy. Like the layperson Bennett, the linguist Cassidy,
to some degree, represented Jamaican as a "dialect" of English, as evidenced in the subtitle of the book: *Three Hundred Years of the English
Language in Jamaica.* In the appendix to the volume Cassidy presented a
consistent, phonemically based writing system for Jamaican Creole.[20] The

orthography was further discussed and illustrated in the introduction to the *Dictionary of Jamaican English,* the name of which confirmed that Jamaican was not an autonomous language but one inseparably linked to English.[21] The Cassidy writing system had the important advantage of not employing any symbols not used in the orthography of English.

In spite of Cassidy's concession to the English writing system, over the years the vast majority of educated literates saw no reason to go to the trouble of learning a new writing system for a set of language varieties that were not "a language" proper. Mervyn Morris, editor of Louise Bennett's *Selected Poems,* gives the commonsense rationale for the writer's choice of an English-looking orthography for Jamaican: "But, anxious not to be rejected unread, most of us have chosen compromise. The most common (if inconsistent) approach is to write the vernacular for the eye accustomed to standard English, but with various alterations signalling creole."[22]

With the strengthening of a mass-based nationalism, alternative views have appeared. For many members of the society, the very difference in the sound values assigned to letters in the Cassidy system makes Jamaican "look" on the page like a language totally distinct from English. For some, this is a deterrent. However, for those wishing to assert the autonomy of a Jamaican national identity, the non-English look of the written language is an advantage. The very strangeness of the orthography restores to Jamaican its integrity; it gives the language and its speakers presence. The "writability" of Jamaican in a coherent, discrete system thus confirms its status as "a language," just like English.

For example, Andrew Sewell, a Jamaican Creole–speaking Rastafarian man, having read a newspaper article written in the Cassidy system, "Cho! Misa Cargill, Riispek Juu!" goes straight to the heart of the matter: "It full [fills] di space of our real African language."[23] The Cassidy orthography, making manifest the languageness of Jamaican Creole, seems to fill the void left by African languages, which have all but disappeared from everyday use in Jamaica. This more positive approach to the Cassidy writing system is relatively recent and certainly not widespread.

294 | Sound Clash

For almost five years, from 1993 to 1998, I (Carolyn) wrote a bilingual English/Jamaican newspaper column for the *Jamaica Observer*.[24] A classic example of the hostile response to this experimental newspaper column is a letter from Sean Reid:

> "It grieves me to take up this newspaper and see the writing of Dr. Carolyn Cooper. It leaves me to ask the question, is Dr. Carolyn Cooper trying to spoil the beautiful English language which we Jamaicans are trying to catch up with?
>
> "The reason why we speak patois is because our forefathers had problems communicating with their slave masters.
>
> "Now that is behind us—and we are moving to a frontier where English is the key language, why then should we go backwards?"[25]

Furthermore, my choice of the Cassidy orthography for the columns written in Jamaican generated even more controversy. In an unpublished paper, "(W)uman Tong(ue): Writing a Bilingual Newspaper Column in 'Post-Colonial' Jamaica," I document the history of the reception of the column, and especially the use of the Jamaican language and the Cassidy orthography on the editorial page of a national newspaper.[26]

There *were* positive responses to the column and to use of the Cassidy orthography. Many readers took pride in their ability to read the ostensibly "difficult" phonetic orthography. One enthusiastic reader gleefully reported that colleagues in her office would crowd around for her to read the Cassidy columns aloud. I found this picture of elitism somewhat disturbing. Advocating mass literacy in Jamaican seemed incompatible with using a specialist orthography that the masses were claiming they could not easily understand. Nevertheless, this vivid image of the reader as the modern equivalent of the oral storyteller engaged in a communal ritual was a reminder of the long tradition in Jamaica of the literate person reading the newspaper—written in English—for attentive listeners. In the spirit of compromise, a dual orthography was later used for the biweekly

Jamaican column, both the Cassidy and the "Chaka-Chaka." That Jamaican Creole word, meaning "disorderly," is of Twi origin—"takataka, muddy, miry"—and accurately denotes the notoriously irregular orthography of English in which the nonspecialist orthographies for Jamaican have their idiosyncratic origins.

Despite considerable resistance to the general use of an efficient writing system for Jamaican, between the 1960s and the present, a small but growing body of Jamaican Creole literature, mainly poetry, has been emerging. A popular sense of national feeling, not to be confused with the elitist kind on which the Jamaican state is based, has been developing quite rapidly among the mass of the population. The speed with which the sense of this alternative national identity has been spreading has quickly outstripped the limited expansion of literature written in Jamaican Creole varieties that has taken place. This popular sense of national identity was crying out for a means of expression in a truly popular body of creative language.

Twentieth-century technology came to the rescue, providing a way around the writing problem. Technologies involving sound amplification—tape recorders, phonograph records, and radio—had made it possible for spoken language to reach much larger audiences than was possible in face-to-face interaction. These technologies did for the spoken word what the printing press had done for writing—multiplied several times over the potential size of the audience for any particular language message. Language transmitted using these technologies, as happened with earlier technologies such as writing and the printing press, came to acquire special status. It is by this means that, with the emergence of radio in Britain, BBC English could come to have at least partly replaced the English of Milton, Shakespeare, and the Bible as the model for standard varieties of British English.

Initially, the new technologies were used to expand the communication network of the elite groups within Jamaica. Soon, however, the elite monopoly of these technologies began to collapse. Radio drama programs

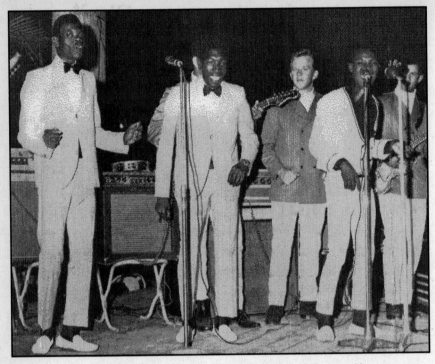

Desmond Dekker and the Aces, winners of the 1968 Festival Song competition, performing at the Governor's Ball, held at King's House. Photo: *Gleaner* Archives, 1968.

and more recently television serials in Jamaican, as well as popular radio talk-shows that give widespread voice to speakers of Jamaican Creole—some bilingual program hosts even speak in Jamaican—have been an important mechanism for developing a truly populist national consciousness.[27]

In addition, in the 1960s, there developed popular local music forms in ska, rock-steady, and reggae. These forms were promoted and popularized through sound amplification, phonograph records, and radio. In the early period, the lyrics of this music were predominantly in language varieties that would be regarded as English or a close approximation thereof. The chorus would often be in some variety of Jamaican. Examples of this kind of song range from "The Israelites" by Desmond Dekker, through "Maccabee Version" by Max Romeo, to "No Woman No Cry" by Bob Marley. An alternative trend involved songs with predominantly Jamaican Creole lyrics, such as "Sweet and Dandy" by the Maytals and "Ramgoat Liver" by Pluto Shervington. Some of the songs of this era were used in the movie *The Harder They Come,* which itself became a "cult" film, replete with English subtitles for foreign audiences unfamiliar with Jamaican, defining for non-Jamaicans as well as Jamaicans the essence of a subversively antiestablishment Jamaican national identity.

Most of this early music was first produced in the recording studio from lyrics that were either improvised or already written. The music thus reached a mass audience primarily through records being played with amplification at dances and in other public places as well as over the radio. Usually after gaining popularity through these media, the music was performed by singers and bands before a live audience. With the appearance of systems of sound amplification that allowed both the recorded music and the disc jockey presenting it to be heard at the same time, the practice developed at dances by the beginning of the 1970s for disc jockeys to do live talking improvisations against the background of recorded music. To facilitate this, the recording studios began to produce reverse sides of 45 rpm records with only the bass and rhythm tracks of the music. Against this musical background, DJs, as they came to be called, would deliver improvised lyrics to live audiences. These lyrics were predominantly in varieties that would be described as Jamaican Creole.

Over time, as is well documented, a new genre developed, known variously as dub, ragga, and dancehall. After multiple presentations in the dancehall to live audiences, particular DJ pieces get recorded and reach a wider audience through cassette tapes, records, compact discs, the radio, and most recently music videos on television. The fact that the riddim is often identical for several DJ tunes confirms the potency of the beat in shaping dancehall aesthetics. The riddim itself becomes a compelling signifier, dubbing several times over the language form and message created by the DJ. The audiences in the dancehall provide instant feed-back, with the DJ, where necessary, adjusting the lyrics in line with the public response. In general, the process of creating and refining a DJ piece is largely oral, with the fixing of the form taking place only when it is eventually recorded. Louise Frazer-Bennett, an icon in her own right—not to be confused with poet and folklorist Louise Bennett—describes the usual creation to performance to recording process:

> The artist may have a punch line or chorus, but not the body of the song. So the engineer, the producer and the artist would collaborate to finish the song. Then the record would be released on test press to the sound systems. In most cases it is the artist who takes the test press to a major dance, uses the B side and does the tune live and bus the place [creates a hit]. After the artist visit four or five major dances with this riddim the producer now gives it to a record distributor who labels the song, gives it to the radio station record library and some of the major disc jockeys. Depending on who the artist and the producer respect, that disc jockey will get first preference to play the tune on the radio.[28]

The DJ phenomenon has helped create an environment in which the production of literature in Jamaican Creole can flourish. A body of poetry has developed that is written to be performed to the same kind of musical accompaniment as that used by DJs. Several dub poets, as they have come to be known, have attracted public attention, and a significant body of dub poetry has emerged. Some of the outstanding poet perform-ers are Linton Kwesi Johnson, Oku Onuora, Jean Breeze, Mikey Smith, and Mutabaruka. Oku Onuora defines "dub poetry" in such a way as to suggest its distance from the conventions of English metrics. It may be written down, but he disclaims any genealogical ties with mainstream English literature: "It's dubbing out the little penta-metre and the little highfalutin business and dubbing in the rootsical, yard, basic rhythm that I-an-I know. Using the language, using the body. It also mean to dub out the isms and schisms and to dub consciousness into the people-dem head. That's dub poetry."[29]

Historian and poet Kamau Brathwaite in his book *History of the Voice,* makes the most precise connection between language and national identity in his coinage of the term "nation language" to define indigenous Caribbean languages such as Jamaican Creole. He argues, somewhat metaphorically like Onuora, "What English has given us as a model for poetry, and to a lesser extent prose (but poetry is the basic tool here), is the pentameter. . . . There have, of course, been attempts to break it."[30] He continues: "It is nation language in the Caribbean that, in fact, largely ignores the pentameter."[31] "Dub poetry" thus marks an important stage in the development of non-elitist nationalist consciousness in Jamaican Creole, among Jamaicans at home, and, equally important, in communities of migrants the world over. However, this material is nowhere as popular nor as much a part of mass consciousness as is mainstream DJ music.

The DJs have produced a significant body of creative language in varieties of Jamaican Creole, not just at home but also in the diaspora.[32] For example, the British based DJ, Macka B, at the December 28, 1991 "Best of White River Reggae Bash" concert in Ocho Rios, recognized the achievements of world-famous Jamaicans who "big-up' the nation," often in "nation language." Citing Marcus Garvey, who is credited with taking black consciousness to African Americans, and Bob Marley who transmitted globally reggae music and Rastafari discourses, sung in the heart language of the Jamaican people, Macka B wittily asserts that Jamaica must have a factory on the island that manufactures cultural nationalists for export. The ironic use of the unexpected metaphor of mechanized production to celebrate the re/production and global dispersal of Jamaican popular culture is a good example of the DJ's characteristically mischievous humor.

Dancehall music has reached a mass audience in Jamaica and other parts of the Caribbean. In addition, it has spread to Jamaican and other Caribbean communities in North America and Europe and expanded into significant sections of the non-Caribbean populations in these countries. It has developed a considerable audience in many countries across the globe. The international recognition being given to this material is acting as a substitute for the validation that would normally come from such material being written down and thus becoming literature. The effect is that the rapidly developing popular national consciousness in Jamaica is moving in the direction of acquiring a language consciousness to accompany it. International interest in the body of creative material produced in the language is fostering the notion of Jamaican Creole as a language separate and apart from all others.

Additional support for this emerging language consciousness is coming from the status and prestige being accorded messages in the electronic media. Radio, television, and the video may be replacing the printed work as the most prestigious medium for transmitting information in language. If this is so, the use of Jamaican Creole in these media can only further enhance the developing prestige of the language, which has latched on to those communication media that are growing in importance. The effect of not having a standard writing system and, hence, a developed body of literature is being minimized.

There is considerable historical precedent for what is happening in the Jamaican situation. States have emerged before as a result of national consciousness triggered by the appearance of an oral rather than a written body of creative material in a language. The oral epics of the *Iliad* and the *Odyssey,* attributed to Homer, formed the bridge between the collapse of the Mycenean Greek state and the reconstitution of a Greek state system some five hundred years later. These oral epics, performed to musical accompaniment in a tradition that seems rather similar to DJ music, formed the basis of preserving the Greek language and national identity over the centuries when no state existed. These epics were a major focal point of national identity when the Greek state was reconstituted. The oral epic has served similar functions among groups as diverse as the Malinke and Songhay of West Africa and among the Serbs and Croats of Yugoslavia.

The developing alternative national identity that has its early origins in maroonage and the traditions of slave resistance is paralleled by complementary developments at other levels of the society. At the level of the economy, there is the development of international trade involving the informal commercial importers. Other economic activities include the cultivation and export of marijuana and the transshipment of cocaine, all defined as illegal by the existing state structure.

There is, as well, the assertion of a mass-based alternative morality as expressed in what the establishment perceives to be the "slack" or vulgar lyrics of much of the DJs' music. Another aspect of this alternative morality is the glorification of gun violence, particularly that employed by gunmen against the forces of law and order, as evidenced in the movie *The Harder They Come*. This celebration of violence is reminiscent of the "heroic" phase that many societies appear to go through in the process of developing state systems.[33] The heroic songs of the Serbs and Croats, the Vedic hymns of ancient India, and the Greek *Iliad* are all works of oral art that glorify violence in pursuit of the national interest. These works serve to justify and legitimate the violence exercised by a national group on others in attempting to achieve its goal of creating a state within secure boundaries. This consolidation of the state, of course, is normally achieved only by military victory over all rivals.

An incipient alternative Jamaican state based on an alternative national identity and national language is decidedly challenging the authority of existing state structures. Since its rival is an existing state within the same physical boundaries, the struggle between the two takes the form of a border clash between the legal and the illegal, between competing moral codes. At the level of language, it manifests itself as a sound clash between English and Jamaican, between a "high" versus a "low" language in a diglossia, and thus, ultimately between a literature and an orature. Jamaican dancehall culture is the megawattage sound system of this new globalized national identity.

Notes

ACKNOWLEDGMENTS

1. First published in Stewart Brown, ed., *The Pressures of the Text: Orality, Texts and the Telling of Tales*, Birmingham: Centre of West African Studies, University of Birmingham, 1995, 60-74.

INTRODUCTION

1. English translation: "Those sound systems are no threat/ They sound as if I'm at home/ Listening to my cassette player." Cocoa Tea, "No Threat," Track 6, *Little Sound Boy,* VP Records. VPCD 1441, 1996.
2. Stuart Hall, "Cultural Studies and the Politics of Internationalization," interview with Kuan-Hsing Chen, in *Stuart Hall: Critical Dialogues in Cultural Studies,* ed. David Morley and Kuan-Hsing Chen, London: Routledge, 1996, 407.
3. The American filmmaker Stephanie Black brilliantly critiques the socioeconomic and cultural impact of globalization on Jamaica in the film *Life and Debt,* Tuff Gong Pictures. 2001. In e-mail correspondence, July 13, 2003, Stephanie reports the following: "After screenings of LIFE AND DEBT, people from all around the world have come up to me and said repeatedly, 'you could have filmed the exact same story in my country'—people from Brazil, people from Ghana, Argentinians—'the IMF situation is, unfortunately, exactly the same, you could have shot it there.' And I say, 'yes, it's true; only then the film wouldn't have had this great reggae soundtrack.'"
4. First published in *Jamaica Journal* 22, 4 (1989): 12-31; 23, 1 (1990): 44-52.
5. I am indebted to Peter Stallybrass and Allon White for the formulation "disgust always bears the imprint of desire." *The Politics and Poetics of Transgression,* Ithaca, N.Y.: Cornell University Press, 1986, 191.
6. Carolyn Cooper, *Noises in the Blood: Orality, Gender and the "Vulgar" Body of Jamaican Popular Culture,* London: Macmillan, 1993, 1994, 2004; Durham, NC: Duke University Press, 1995, 2000, 136-173.
7. Ibid., 174.
8. Cary Nelson, Paula A. Treichler, and Lawrence Grossberg, eds., *Cultural Studies,* New York: Routledge, 1992, 13.
9. Norman Stolzoff, *Wake the Town and Tell the People: Dancehall Culture in Jamaica,* Durham, NC: Duke University Press, 2000, 18-19.
10. Mark Cummings, "I have learnt my lesson—*Sean Paul,*" *Daily Observer,* August 13, 2003, 25.
11. Anthony B, "Nah Vote Again," Track 7, *Universal Struggle,* VP Records, VPCD 1510 2, 1997.
12. Carolyn Cooper, *Noises in the Blood,* 4-5.

13. Ibid., 138.

14. Stolzoff, *Wake the Town and Tell the People*, 266.

15. William Henry, "Reggae/Dancehall Music as an Autonomous Space for Cultural Expression," B.A. dissertation, Goldsmiths College, London University, 1997, 25.

16. Ibid., 26.

17. Ibid., 27.

18. Ibid.

19. Cooper, *Noises in the Blood*, 136.

20. Ibid., 139.

21. Ibid., 172.

22. Henry, "Reggae/Dancehall Music," 26-27. Henry reproduced this argument in a 2001 public lecture at the University of the West Indies, Mona, hosted by the Reggae Studies Centre.

23. Iris Myrie, "Distasteful Side of Dancehall Music," *Gleaner*, February 14, 2003, A5.

24. Ibid.

25. Sugar Minott, "Can't Cross The Border," Track 7, *Little Sound Boy*, VP Records, VPCD 1441, 1996. Regrettably, permission to reproduce the song here has not been successfully negotiated.

26. Ibid.

27. Tony Rebel, "Chatty Chatty," Track 9, *Just Ragga*, Charm Records, CRCD14, 1992.

28. Ibid.

29. Ibid.

30. Ibid.

31. Ibid.

32. Ibid.

33. In the eastern Caribbean, dancehall is known as dub, and in the United Kingdom it is known as ragga. I am indebted to Moses "Beenie Man" Davis for the insight that what is termed "dancehall" music should more appropriately be called "rub a dub" music. In conversation, February 26, 2003.

34. Ian Boyne, "'Bling-Bling Christianity Run Things," *Sunday Gleaner*, July 20, 2003, G2.

35. David Scott, "'Wi a di Govament': An Interview with Anthony B," *Small Axe* 2 (September 1997): 100. The structure of Anthony B's language seems more English than Jamaican in this interview. Though politically incorrect, I change the orthography from the specialized Cassidy system for the Jamaican language used by David Scott, "anglicizing" it in order to facilitate readability. I translate, in brackets, the distinctly Jamaican vocabulary and syntax.

36. Ibid.

37. Ibid.

38. Stolzoff, *Wake the Town and Tell the People*, 267.

39. Carolyn Cooper, "Slackness Hiding From Culture: Erotic Play in the Dancehall," in *Noises in the Blood*, 142-43.

40. Ibid., 162-63.

41. Ibid., 164-65.

42. Ibid., 148.

43. Ibid.

44. Stolzoff, *Wake the Town and Tell the People*, 267-68.

45. Buju Banton, "Boom Bye Bye." Track 1, *Strictly the Best,* Vol. 9, VP Records, VPCD 1291, 1993.
46. Carolyn Cooper, "'Lyrical Gun': Metaphor and Role Play in Jamaican Dancehall Culture," *The Massachusetts Review* 35, 3-4 (1994): 447.
47. Andrew Ross, "Mr. Reggae DJ, Meet the International Monetary Fund," in *Real Love: In Pursuit of Cultural Justice* (New York: New York University Press, 1998), 60.
48. Ibid., 60-61.
49. Cooper, "'Lyrical Gun,'"447.
50. Ross, "Mr. Reggae DJ, Meet the International Monetary Fund," 61.
51. Cooper, "'Lyrical Gun,'" 440.
52. Ibid., 59.
53. Ibid., 439.
54. Stolzoff, *Wake the Town and Tell the People,* 19.
55. Ibid.
56. Ibid., xiv.
57. Jamaica Kincaid, *Lucy,* New York: Farrar Straus and Giroux, 1990, 56.
58. Corneldi Watts, "Ban the Nasty Lyrics," *Barbados Advocate,* June 23, 2002, 11. I looked up Watts's number in the telephone directory but she was not listed. I would have enjoyed talking with her on the matter.

CHAPTER 1

1. Ninjaman, "Border Clash," Track 4, Side Two, *Warning You Now,* Jammy$ Records, 1990. The song is worthy of much more ample quotation but because permission to reproduce it here has not been successfully negotiated, I have had to resort to paraphrase in the analysis below.
2. Donna Hope, "Inna Di Dancehall Dis/place: Socio-Cultural Politics of Identity in Jamaica," Master's of Philosophy thesis, University of the West Indies, Mona, 2001, 146-47.
3. Ibid., 147-48.
4. Ninjaman, in telephone conversation with me, August 10, 2002.
5. Ninjaman, in telephone conversation with me, August 10, 2002.
6. Ras Dizzy, a talented intuitive painter whose work has been exhibited in art galleries in Jamaica and overseas and reproduced in books, wrote occasional letters that were distributed on the campus of the University of the West Indies, Mona. The one from which I quote is dated April 18, 1971. Ras Dizzy still sells paintings on the Mona campus more than three decades later.
7. *Weekend Observer,* March 6, 1998, 4.
8. Denise Noble, "Ragga Music: Dis/Respecting Black Women and Dis/Reputable Sexualities," in Barnor Hesse, ed., *Un/settled Multiculturalisms: Diasporas, Entanglements, Transruptions,* London: Zed Books, 2000, 151.
9. Thanks to Professor Hubert Devonish, Department of Language, Linguistics and Philosophy, University of the West Indies, Mona, Jamaica, for clarification of the "folk etymology" argument outlined below.
10. Shabba Ranks, "Back and Bellyrat," Track 4, *Just Reality,* Vine Yard Records, VYDCD 6, 1991.

11. Terror Fabulous, "Praise Jah & Live," Track 2, *Kette Drum*, Digital B, DBCD 2039, n.d.
12. *The Guardian*, December 8, 1995, 14.
13. Ibid.
14. Ibid.
15. We borrow this clever turn of phrase from the title of a book fleetingly glimpsed in a London bookshop for which we do not have the reference.
16. "Free Thinker," "Right to Hold an Opinion," *Gleaner*, March 8, 1993, 7.
17. George Lipsitz, *Dangerous Crossroads: Popular Music, Postmodernism and the Poetics of Place*, London: Verso, 1994, 5.
18. Buju Banton, "Deportees (Things Change)," Track 4, *Voice of Jamaica*, Mercury, 518 013-2, 1993.
19. Julian Cowell, "Jamaicans in U.S. Prisons," *Abeng Newsletter* 3, 1 (January-March 1998): 10.
20. Winston James, "Migration, Racism and Identity Formation: The Caribbean Experience in Britain," in Winston James and Clive Harris, eds., *Inside Babylon: The Caribbean Diaspora in Britain*, London: Verso, 1993, 245-46.
21. There are two dimensions to this: the comic one of the Jamaican interpretation of returnees from the United Kingdom, as "maddy maddy," not least because of the brisk, nontropical pace at which they walk. The second dimension is more tragic: There is a substantial literature discussing the violence that a racist Britain wreaks on the mental health of Caribbean migrants. See, for example, Errol Francis, "Psychiatric Racism and Social Police: Black People and the Psychiatric Services," in James and Harris, eds., *Inside Babylon*, 179-205.
22. Richard Burton, *Afro-Creole: Power, Opposition and Play in the Caribbean*, Ithaca, NY: Cornell University Press, 1997, 6.
23. For an elaboration of this argument, see Carolyn Cooper, "Slackness Hiding from Culture: Erotic Play in the Dancehall," in *Noises in the Blood*, 136-173.
24. This theme is elaborated in the February 2002 Bob Marley lecture entitled "'Incline Thine Ear': Roots, Reality and Culture in Jamaican Dancehall DJ Music," given by Cecil Gutzmore at the University of the West Indies, Mona.
25. Anthony B, "One Thing," Track 3, *Real Revolutionary*, Greensleeves, GRELCD 230, 1996; apparently issued as *So Many Things* by VP in the United States.
26. David Scott, "'Wi a di Govament': An Interview with Anthony B.," *Small Axe* 2 (September 1997): 88.
27. Anthony B, "Fire Pon Rome," Track 8, *Real Revolutionary*, Greensleeves, GRELCD230, 1996.
28. Jamaican cultural analyst and radio talk-show host Tony Laing also makes this point on an "Impact" talk-show program focusing on dancehall culture, hosted by Cliff Hughes on CVM Televsion and first broadcast on November 24, 2002.
29. Edward Baugh, *It Was the Singing*, Toronto & Kingston: Sandberry Press, 2000, 74.
30. David Scott, "'Wi a di Govament,'" 83. Bobo is Richard Bell, Anthony B's manager.
31. Anthony B, "Nah Vote Again," Track 7, *Universal Struggle*, VP Records, VPCD 1510 2, 1997.
32. Louise Bennett, *Jamaica Labrish*, Kingston: Sangster's, 1966, 131-32.
33. Ibid., 134
34. Scott, "'Wi a di Govament,'" 85.

35. Ibid.
36. Anthony B, "Swarm Me," Track 10, *Real Revolutionary*, Greensleeves, GRELCD230, 1996.
37. Scott, "'Wi a di Govament,'" 93.
38. Ibid., 92.
39. Anthony B, "Marley Memories," Track 16, *Universal Struggle*, VP Records, VPCD 1510 2, 1997.
40. Scott, "'Wi a di Govament,'" 91.
41. Ibid, 88.
42. Buju Banton, "I.C.I.," Track 4, *Cell Block, Vol. 2*, Penthouse Records, CBCD2032, 1995. Regrettably, permission to reproduce the song here has not been successfully negotiated.
43. Claude McKay, "The Apple Woman's Complaint," published in Wayne F. Cooper, ed. *The Passion of Claude McKay: Selected Poetry and Prose, 1912-1948*, New York: Schocken Books, 1973, 112-13.
44. Vernon Davidson, "Charles Offers Solution to Street Vending Problem," *Daily Observer*, January 1, 2003, 3.
45. Ibid.

CHAPTER 2

1. The meaning of the Jamaican word *liriks* is somewhat wider than the English "lyrics." In Jamaican, *liriks* functions as both noun and verb. It generalizes the singer's skill with lyrics into any kind of verbal skill and especially refers to the language of seduction.
2. Tom Willis, "From Ragga to Riches," *Sunday Times* (London), April 4, 1993.
3. Ibid.
4. Andrew Clunis, "Banned: London pressures dancehall stars," *The Sunday Gleaner*, June 27, 2004, A1.
5. For a fuller reading of Marley's corpus of song texts, see "Chanting Down Babylon: Bob Marley's Song as Literary Text," in Carolyn Cooper, *Noises in the Blood*, 117-35, and, more recently, Kwame Dames, *Bob Marley: Lyrical Genius*, 2002.
6. Bob Marley, "Bad Card," Track 3, *Uprising*, Tuff Gong Records, 422-846 211-2, 1980.
7. Peter Tosh, "Equal Rights," Track 5, *Equal Rights*, CBS Records, CK 34670, 1977.
8. Bob Marley, "Bad Card."
9. Beenie Man, "Slam," Track 2, *Blessed*, Island Records, IJCD 3005/524 138-2, 1995.
10. Bob Marley, "Kinky Reggae," Track 7, *Catch a Fire*, Tuff Gong Records, 422-846 201-2, 1973.
11. "Rent-a-tile" refers to the small space on the dance floor that would accommodate dancers locked in a tight embrace.
12. Beres Hammond, "Rock Away," Track 5, *Music Is Life*, VP Records, VPCD1624, 2001.
13. Ibid.
14. Ibid.
15. Ibid.

16. Ibid.
17. The symposium was organized by political philosopher Dr. Clinton Hutton of the Department of Government, University of the West Indies, Mona. The derogatory expression, "nasty nayga," my distillation of Gloudon's argument, is equivalent to the American racial slur, "filthy nigger." The exchange between myself and Mrs. Gloudon is reported inaccurately by a freelance writer with an entirely appropriate pseudonym, "Chaos." See "Question and Answer Session Turns Passionate," *Gleaner*, May 15, 2002, C3.
18. Ninjaman, "Test the High Power," Track 2, *Little Sound Boy*, VP Records, VPCD1441, 1996. Regrettably, permission to reproduce the song here has not been successfully negotiated.
19. Shabba Ranks, "Just Reality," Track 6, *Rough & Ready Vol. 1*, Sony 471442 2, 1992. Regrettably, permission to reproduce the song here has not been successfully negotiated.
20. Bob Marley, "Waiting in Vain," Track 7, *Exodus*, Tuff Gong Records, 422-846 208-2, 1977.
21. Bob Marley, "Pimper's Paradise," Track 7, *Uprising*, Tuff Gong Records, 422-846 211-2, 1980.
22. Ibid.
23. Ibid.
24. Ibid.
25. Shabba Ranks, "Ca'an Dun," Track 8, *Rough & Ready*, Vol. 1, Sony 471442 2, 1992.
26. Shabba Ranks, "Gone Up," Track 5, *As Raw as Ever*, Sony, 468102 2, 1991.
27. Ibid.
28. Ibid.
29. Ibid.
30. Ibid.
31. Louise Bennett, *Aunty Roachy Seh*, ed. Melvin Morris, Kingston: Sangster's, 1993, 67.
32. Ian Boyne, "True and Still Unspoilt Icon: The One and Only Miss Lou," *Sunday Gleaner*, August 3, 2003, G3.
33. Louise Bennett, *Selected Poems*, ed. Mervyn Morris, Kingston: Sangster's, 1982, 58.
34. Ibid., 142.
35. Shabba Ranks, "Gone Up," Track 5, *As Raw as Ever*, Sony, 468102 2, 1991.
36. Shabba Ranks, "Woman Tangle," Track 3, *As Raw as Ever*, Sony, 468102 2, 1991.
37. The *Daily Observer* of December 31, 2002, carried a front-page report headlined "Children's Homes Review Ordered: Study to Determine if Ja Meeting UN Child Rights Obligations."
38. Shabba Ranks, "Park Yu Benz," Track 12, *As Raw as Ever*, Sony 468102 2, 1991.
39. Ibid.
40. Shabba Ranks, "Flesh Axe," Track 7, *As Raw as Ever*, Sony, 468102 2, 1991.
41. "Batty rider" means, approximately, "shorts that ride high on the bottom."
42. Lisa Jones, *Bulletproof Diva: Tales of Race, Sex, and Hair*, New York: Doubleday, 1994, 74.
43. See proverb 7, cited below.
44. Shabba Ranks, "Muscle Grip," Track, *X-Tra Naked*, Sony Epic, EK 52464, 1992.

45. "According to the *Dictionary of Jamaican* English, a 'coco-head' is the rootstock or rhizome of the coco plant as distinct from the tuber, which is a coco."
46. A *bankra* basket, normally larger than the "cutacoo."
47. A *cutacoo* is a field basket used by hunters and cultivators.
48. Here literal "firewood," which denotes material prosperity, becomes a metaphor for the erect penis: "wood" as "hood."

CHAPTER 3

1. Luisah Teish, "Daughter of Promise: Oriki Oshun," *Carnival of the Spirit*, San Francisco: Harper, 1994, 75.
2. Obiagele Lake, *Rastafari Women: Subordination in the Midst of Liberation Theology*, Durham: Carolina Academic Press, 1998, 131.
3. Lady Saw, "Stab Out Mi Meat," *The Collection*, Diamond Rush, DRCD 003, 1997.
4. Lake appears to use as the text of the song Lady Saw's abbreviated performance on the Isaac Julien film, *The Darker Side of Black*, in which the DJ does say "Stab up mi meat."
5. Female DJ Ce'Cile in her song "Do It To Me" celebrates the pleasures of cunnilingus, advising men to speak the truth about their sexual practices: "Watch dem a talk bout no but dem a dweet" [Just look at them saying no but they do it], King of Kings label, 2003.
6. Lake's transcription is inaccurate: "outa street" [out on the streets] becomes the nonsensical "out of straight." In performance, Lady Saw elongates the vowel so that 'street' does sound like 'straight.' But knowledge of the language makes the meaning clear.
7. Obiagele Lake, *Rastafari Women: Subordination in the Midst of Liberation Theology*, Durham: Carolina Academic Press, 1998, 132.
8. Carolyn Cooper, interview in Isaac Julien, *The Darker Side of Black*.
9. Ibid.
10. Lake, *Rastafari Women*, 132.
11. Ibid., 132-33.
12. Ibid., 79.
13. For this insight I am indebted to L'Antoinette Stines, Yoruba priestess, artistic director of the L'ACADCO Dance Company, and a Ph.D. candidate in Cultural Studies at the University of the West Indies, Mona. The Dictionary of Jamaican English defines "myal" thus: "cf Hausa maye, 1. Sorcerer, wizard; 2. Intoxication; Return. (All of these senses are present in the Jamaican use of the word.) . . . . In recent use in AFRICAN and similar cults: formal possession by the spirit of a dead ancestor, and the dance done under possession." An alternative etymology for "myal"—which admits moral ambivalence—is provided by the linguist Hazel Carter in personal communication with Maureen Warner-Lewis, March 1985: "mayal < Mayaala, Kikongo, 'person/thing exercising control.'"
14. Cited in Frederic Cassidy, *Jamaica Talk*, Basingstoke and London: Institute of Jamaica/Macmillan, 1961, 184.
15. Ibid, 252.
16. Bibi Bakere-Yusuf, e-mail correspondence with author, January 13, 2003.

17. Oyeronke Oyewumi, *The Invention of Women: Making an African Sense of Western Gender Discourses*, Minneapolis: University of Minnesota Press, 1997, 174.
18. Ibid.
19. Teish, *Carnival of the Spirit*, 79-80.
20. Shabba Ranks, "Flesh Axe," Track 7, *As Raw as Ever*, Sony, 468102 2, 1991.
21. Peter Tosh, interviewed by Carolyn Cooper, *Pulse* (June 1984): 12.
22. Donald Hogg, "The Convince Cult in Jamaica," *Yale University Publications in Anthropology* 58: 4. Reprinted in Sidney Mintz, comp., *Papers in Caribbean Anthropology*, New Haven: Human Relations Area Files Press, 1970. I am indebted to Burton Sankeralli, a graduate student in Cultural Studies at the University of the West Indies, Mona, for bringing these pum-pum references to my attention, via Cecil Gutzmore.
23. Ibid., 11
24. Ibid.
25. Maureen Warner-Lewis, *Central Africa in the Caribbean: Transcending Time, Transforming Cultures*. Kingston, Jamaica: University of the West Indies Press, 2003, 235-36.
26. Prezident Brown and Don Yute, "African Ting," Track 10, *Prezident Selections*, RUNNetherlands, RNN0043, n.d.
27. Papa Pilgrim, "Reggae Sunsplash 93: Report From Yard," *The Beat* 12, 5 (1993): 49.
28. Lady Saw, "What Is Slackness," Track 2, *Give Me the Reason*, Diamond Rush, RUSHCD1, 1996.
29. Lady Saw, "Bun Mi Out," 45 rpm, Diamond Rush, 1994.
30. Lady Saw, "Glory Be to God," Track 6, *Give Me the Reason*, Diamond Rush, RUSHCD1, 1996.
31. Lady Saw, "Condom," Track 9, *Give Me the Reason*, Diamond Rush, RUSHCD1, 1996.
32. Ibid.
33. Ibid.
34. Ibid.
35. Ibid.
36. Ibid.
37. Ibid.

CHAPTER 4

1. Sandra Lee, interviewed on Anthony Miller's "Entertainment Report," broadcast on Television Jamaica, April 23, 1999. Donna Hope describes Sandra Lee thus in her Master's dissertation, "Inna Di Dancehall Dis/place: Socio-cultural Politics of Identity in Jamaica," University of the West Indies, Mona, 2001, 91: "She lays claim to a legacy of urban, inner-city/downtown Kingston background and higgler/ dancehall heritage that places her in a position of royalty in the dancehall dis/place. Her arrival at any dancehall event, major, minor or otherwise is heralded by an announcement over the sound system and her high status in the dancehall dis/place

is consistently re-presented and legitimized by the consistent symbolizing and legitimizing of her presence at this event."

2. *Dancehall Queen*, Dirs. Don Letts & Rick Elgood, Island Jamaica Films, Island Digital Media, 1997.

3. A personal anecdote will illustrate the point: One of my former students at the University of the West Indies, who works at an upmarket car sales company, tried unsuccessfully to get me to trade in my entirely trustworthy Honda Accord for an Audi A4. One of her "compelling" arguments was that I would look so good in the car. I managed to convince her that, for me, a car is not primarily a fashion accessory.

4. Maggie Humm, "Is the Gaze Feminist? Pornography, Film and Feminism" in Gary Day and Clive Bloom, eds., *Perspectives on Pornography: Sexuality in Film and Literature*, London: Macmillan, 1988, 70-71.

5. Ibid., 71.

6. Walter Jekyll, ed., *Jamaican Song and Story*, London: David Nutt, 1907, xxxvi.

7. Ibid, xxxvii.

8. Ibid.

9. "Picky-picky head" is a derogatory Jamaican Creole expression. The *Dictionary of Jamaican English* cites the following 1960 usage: "when a girl's hair is very short, grows close to the scalp in little balls of fluff, very negroid."

10. Ingrid Banks, *Hair Matters: Beauty Power, and Black Consciousness*, New York: New York University Press, 2000, 69.

11. Catherine Constable, "Making Up the Truth: On Lies, Lipstick and Friedrich Nietzsche," in Stella Bruzzi and Pamela Church Gibson, eds., *Fashion Cultures: Theories, Explorations and Analysis*, London: Routledge, 2000, 191.

12. Ibid., 199.

13. Banks, *Hair Matters*, 3.

14. Cornel West, *Race Matters*, Boston: Beacon Press, 1993, 85.

15. Buchi Emecheta, *The Joys of Motherhood*, 1979; rpt London: Heinemann, 1980, 71.

16. For this anecdote, I am indebted to Professor Hubert Devonish, Department of Language, Linguistics & Philosophy at the University of the West Indies, Mona, Jamaica. A rough translation of the verse: "For figure and face I didn't place; but for boobs and arse I busted their arse."

17. Greg Tate, *Flyboy in the Buttermilk: Essays on Contemporary America*, New York: Fireside Simon & Schuster, 1992, 95.

18. Ibid.

19. Bibi Bakere-Yusuf in e-mail correspondence with me, January 10, 2003.

20. Frantz Fanon, *Black Skin, White Masks*, 1952; rpt New York: Grove Press, 1967, 111.

21. Bakere-Yusuf in e-mail correspondence with me.

22. The etymology of "mampi," which does not appear in the *Dictionary of Jamaican English*, is obscure. It means full-figured.

23. Buju Banton, "Gal You Body Good," Track 1, *Buju Banton Meets Garnett Silk and Tony Rebel at the Super Stars Conference*, Rhino Records, RNCD 2033 n.d.

24. The Dictionary of Jamaican English defines "maaga" as "[t]hin, lean; by implication, often underfed, half-starved."

25. *Babymother*, Dir. Julian Henriques, Formation Films, Film Four Distributors, 1998.

26. Olive Senior, *Arrival of the Snake-Woman and Other Stories*, London: Longman Caribbean, 1989, 121.

CHAPTER 5

1. Ian Boyne, "How Dancehall Promotes Violence," *Sunday Gleaner*, December 22, 2002, G1.
2. Ian Boyne, "How Dancehall Holds Us Back," *Sunday Gleaner*, December 29, 2002, G1.
3. Ibid.
4. Melville Cooke, "Ninja Man, Reneto Adams—Both above the Law," *Gleaner*, January 3, 2003, A4.
5. Pan Head and Sugar Black, "A Wi Run the Gun Them," Track 20, *Buju Banton Meets Garnett Silk and Tony Rebel at the Super Stars Conference*, Rhino Records Ltd., n.d., RNCD 2033.
6. Ibid.
7. Ibid. The word, in the original Dennis Brown song is "oppression," not "pressure."
8. Boyne, "How Dancehall Promotes Violence," G3.
9. Cooke, "Ninja Man, Reneto Adams."
10. Spragga Benz and Elephant Man, "Warrior Cause," Track 6, *Strictly the Best*, Volume 27, VP Records, VPCD1639, 2001.
11. I am indebted to Sean Mock Yen of the Radio Education Unit, University of the West Indies, Mona, for the transcription of the song text.
12. Monty Alexander, "Cowboys Talk," Track 5, *Caribbean Circle*, Chesky Records, JD80, 1992.
13. Bob Marley interview with Dermott Hussey, Track 20, *Talkin' Blues*, Tuff Gong Records, 422-848 243-2, 1991.
14. Michael Thelwell, *The Harder They Come*, London: Pluto, 1980, 221.
15. Shabba Ranks, "Gun Pon Me," Track 4, *As Raw as Ever*, Epic Records, EK 47310, 1991.
16. Ibid.
17. Ibid.
18. Ibid.
19. The Ethiopians, "Gun Man," Track 12, *The Ethiopians*, Trojan Records, CDTRL 228, 1988; 1986.
20. Robert Carr, "On 'Judgements': Poverty, Sexuality-Based Violence and Human Rights in 21st Century Jamaica," *The Caribbean Journal of Social Work* 2 (July 2003): 82.
21. TOK, "Chi-Chi Man," Track 4, *Reggae Gold 2001*, VP Records, VPCD 1629, 2001.
22. Hilary Standing, "Aids: Conceptual and Methodological Issues in Researching Sexual Behaviour in Sub-Saharan Africa," *Social Science Medicine* 34, 5 (1992): 475-76.
23. Ibid., 480.
24. Ibid.
25. Ibid.
26. Ibid.

27. Al Creighton, "Race, Culture and 'Dirty Music,'" *Stabroek News*, September 13, 1992, 15.
28. Lickmout Lou, "Sodom an' Gomorrah right hey!" *Barbados Advocate*, November 6, 1992, 9.
29. Ibid.
30. As an analyst of Jamaican popular culture, I was invited to exchange ideas with Donald Suggs, a representative of GLAAD, on a local radio program, "The Breakfast Club."
31. Ransdell Pierson, "'Kill Gays' Hit Song Stirs Fury," *New York Post*, October 24-25, 1992, 5.
32. I am indebted to Cordell Green, chairman of the Broadcasting Commission, for his assistance in providing data documenting the controversy.
33. Ibid.
34. Cordell Green, e-mail correspondence, June 11, 2003.
35. Peter Noel, "Batty Boys in Babylon," *Village Voice,* January 12, 1993.
36. Pierson, "'Kill Gays' Hit Song Stirs Fury."
37. *Fleg* seems to be related to the English "flag," as in the *Oxford English Dictionary* definition "to lag through fatigue; to lose vigour or energy."
38. Buju Banton, "Have to Get You Tonight," Track 6, *Mr Mention*, Polygram Records, 522 022–2, 1994.
39. John Rashford, "Plants, Spirits and the Meaning of 'John' in Jamaica", *Jamaica Journal* 17, 2 (1984): 62.
40. Edward Long, *The History of Jamaica*, 1774; rpt London: Frank Cass, 1970, Vol. 2, 424.
41. "Mr Nine" is coauthored with Gregory Isaacs.
42. Buju Banton, "Murderer," Track 3, *'Til Shiloh*, Loose Cannon, 314-524 119-2, 1995.
43. Extracted from a longer version of chapter 1, "Border Clash: Sites of Contestation," in which Gutzmore gives a detailed critique of Andrew Ross's dismissive reading of "Murderer" as, first, "censorious" and later, "quite conventional;" the former appears in Ross's paper, "The Structural Adjustment Blues," 1; and the latter in "Mr. Reggae DJ, Meet the International Monetary Fund," in *Real Love: In Pursuit of Cultural Justice*, New York: New York University Press, 1998, 41.
44. Buju Banton, "Mr Nine," Track 19, *Friends for Life*, VP Records/Atlantic, 0 7567 83634 2, 2003. Regrettably, permission to reproduce the song here has not been successfully negotiated.
45. Michael Conally, "Defen' it," *Pure Class*, the *Jamaica Herald*'s Sunday magazine, November 29, 1992, 12.

CHAPTER 6

1. Balford Henry, "Bob and Bounty," *Weekend Star*, February 5, 1999, 23.
2. Bounty Killer, "Sufferah," Track 2, *Ghetto Dictionary: The Mystery*, VP Records, VPCD 1681, 2002.
3. Patricia Meschino, "The Marley Brothers Shining Sons," *Rhythm Magazine*, 86 (June 2000): 27.
4. Ibid.

5. Ibid.
6. Ibid.
7. "War," Track 9, *Rastaman Vibration*, Tuff Gong Records, 422-846 205-2, 1976.
8. Mark Fineman, "Attack Points to 'Lethal' Mix of Religion, Rebellion, Drugs." *Los Angeles Times*, January 7, 2001, A1.
9. Ibid.
10. Ibid.
11. Ibid.
12. Ibid.
13. Bob Marley, "Talkin' Blues," Track 8, *Natty Dread*, Tuff Gong Records, 422-846 204-2, 1974.
14. Ibid.
15. Bob Marley, "One Love/People Get Ready," Track 10, *Exodus*, Tuff Gong Records, 422-846 208-2.
16. Ibid.
17. Dawn Ritch, "Tourism Madness," *Sunday Gleaner*, January 13, 1991, 8A.
18. Rex Nettleford, "War, Recession and Gorillas (Tourism Madness Indeed!)," *Sunday Gleaner*, January 16, 1991, 19B.
19. Ibid.
20. Jamaica Tourist Board television commercial.
21. Bob Marley, "One Drop," Track 7, *Survival*, Tuff Gong Records, 422-846 202-2, 1979.
22. Bob Marley, "Burnin' and Lootin'," Track 4, *Burnin'*, Tuff Gong Records, 422-846 200-2, 1973.
23. Niney, "Blood and Fire," Track 15, *Reggae Hit the Town*, CD 2, *Tougher than Tough: The Story of Jamaican Music*, Island Records, CD2 518 401-2, 1993.
24. Steve Barrow, *Tougher Than Tough: 35 Years of Jamaican Hits*, Island Records Box Set, 1993, 42.
25. Alexander Cruden, *Complete Concordance to the Old and New Testament*, London: Frederick Warne, 3rd edition, 1769, 166.
26. Ibid.
27. Bob Marley, "Revolution," Track 9, *Natty Dread*.
28. Ibid.
29. Ibid.
30. Ibid.
31. Bob Marley, "Ride Natty Ride," Track 8, *Survival*.
32. Ibid.
33. Courtney Walsh, an international cricket star, is a Jamaican fast bowler of legendary speed.
34. Both Marley references are inaccurate, anglicized transcriptions: "table have turned" becomes "tables have turned" and "mek i bun" becomes "mek it bun." The transcriptions hover on the edge of translation.
35. Capleton, "Fire Chant," Track 1, *More Fire*, VP Records, VPCD 1587, 2000.
36. Ibid.
37. Bob Marley, "Ambush in the Night," Track 9, *Survival*.
38. Capleton, "I Am," Track 1, *One Mission*, J & D Distributors, JDCD 0013, 1999.
39. Capleton, "More Prophet," Track 7, *More Fire*, VP Records, VPCD 1587, 2000.
40. Capleton, "Hunt You," Track 8, *More Fire*, VP Records, VPCD 1587, 2000.

41. Ibid.
42. Ibid.
43. Ibid.
44. Bob Marley, "Who the Cap Fit," Track 7, *Rastaman Vibration*, Tuff Gong Records, 422-846 205-2, 1976.
45. Ibid.
46. Bob Marley, "Babylon System," Track 4, *Survival*.
47. Ibid.

CHAPTER 7

1. Curwen Best, "Caribbean Music and the Discourse of AIDS," *Small Axe*, No. 3, March 1998, 57.
2. Gordon Rohlehr, "Folk Research: Fossil or Living Bone?," *The Massachusetts Review*, Autumn-Winter 1994, 392.
3. David Ellis, "Talk Caribbean" television program, Caribbean Broadcasting Union, April 9, 2000.
4. Jamaica Kincaid, *Annie John*, New York: Farrar Straus and Giroux, 1983, 79-80.
5. Gordon Rohlehr, "Folk Research: Fossil or Living Bone?" *Massachusetts Review* (Autumn-Winter 1994): 392.
6. Ibid.
7. "Vile Vocals: Unofficial War in Bim," *Barbados Advocate*, April 11, 2000, 8.
8. Nathaniel Mackey, "An Interview with Kamau Brathwaite," in Stewart Brown, ed., *The Art of Kamau Brathwaite*, Mid Glamorgan: Seren, 1995, 29-30.
9. "Vile Vocals: Unofficial War in Bim."
10. In conversation with me; reproduced in Carolyn Cooper, "Race and the Cultural Politics of Self-Representation: A View from the University of the West Indies," *Research in African Literatures* 27, 4 (1996): 100.
11. Bob Marley, "Redemption Song," Track 10, *Uprising*, Tuff Gong Records, ILPS 9596, 1980.
12. Bob Marley, "Babylon System," Track 4, *Survival*, Island Records, 422-846 211-2, 1979.
13. The University of the West Indies was first established as a college of the University of London in 1948.
14. Carolyn Cooper, "War on Ignorance," *Sunday Advocate*, April 16, 2001, 13.
15. Back cover blurb, George Lamming, *In the Castle of My Skin*, rpt London: Longman, Caribbean, 1992; reprint of Michael Joseph, 1953.
16. Ibid., 287.
17. Barbara Lalla, *Defining Jamaican Fiction: Marronage and the Discourse of Survival*, Tuscaloosa: University of Alabama Press, 1996, 174-75.
18. Ibid.
19. "Bad Product: Don't Import the Garbage," *Barbados Advocate*, April 10, 2000, 8.
20. Ibid.
21. *Sunshine*, April 9, 2000, 2.
22. *Weekend Nation*, April 14, 2000, 9.
23. Adonijah, "Dub's Not the Force of All Evil," *Weekend Nation*, April 14, 2000, 13
24. Ibid.

25. Ibid.

26. In a front-page story on April 11, 2000, headlined "Bottle Ban: Strict Rules for Kensington," the *Barbados Advocate* reports that "[f]ollowing last year's bottle-throwing incident at Kensington Oval, the Barbados Cricket Association has outlawed the bringing of any kind of glass bottle on to the premises at any time before, during or after play."

27. "Bad Product: Don't Import the Garbage."

28. CARICOM, the Caribbean Community, was established in 1973 to foster integration among the small-island states of the Anglophone Caribbean. The Community now includes Haiti and Suriname.

CHAPTER 8

1. Kamau Brathwaite, *"Jah," The Arrivants: A New World Trilogy*, Oxford: Oxford University Press, rpt. 1978, 162. Subsequent references are cited in the text.

2. For a characteristically brilliant reading, see Gordon Rohlehr's analysis of Brathwaite's use of musical allusion in the poem in "Bridges of Sound: An Approach to Edward Brathwaite's 'Jah,'" *Caribbean Quarterly*, 26, 1-2 (1980): 13-31.

3. For a classic account of the role of Harlem as a meeting place of dispersed African peoples, see Claude McKay's *Home to Harlem* 1928; rpt Chatham: Chatham Bookseller, 1973.

4. Fernando Gonzalez, liner notes to Danilo Perez, *Central Avenue*, Impulse, IMCD 279, 1998.

5. Garth White, "Traditional Musical Practice in Jamaica and Its Influence on the Birth of Modern Jamaican Popular Music," African-Caribbean Institute of Jamaica monograph, 64-65, extracted from *ACIJ Newsletter* 7 (March 1982).

6. Linton Kwesi Johnson, introduction to *Tougher Than Tough The Story of Jamaican Music*, Island Records Box Set, 1993, 5.

7. Ben Mapp, "First Reggae. Then Rap. Now It's Dancehall," *New York Times*, June 21, 1992, 23.

8. I am indebted to the Center for African American Studies (CAAS), Institute of American Studies, UCLA, where much of the early work for this chapter was done while on a research fellowship in 1996.

9. I am indebted to Professor Hubert Devonish, Department of Language and Linguistics, University of the West Indies, Mona, for this insight.

10. Stephen Davis, *Reggae Bloodlines: In Search of the Music and Culture of Jamaica*, 1977; rpt London: Heinemann Educational Books, 1981, 17.

11. Mandingo, "The Origins and Meanings of Dancehall & Ragamuffin," *Dance Hall* 1, 1 (February 1994): 14.

12. Ibid.

13. Raquel Rivera, *New York Ricans from the Hip Hop Zone*, New York: Palgrave Macmillan, 2003, 51-52.

14. Marshall Berman, *All That Is Solid Melts into Air*, New York: Simon & Schuster, 1982, 290-92, cited in Tricia Rose, *Black Noise: Rap Music and Black Culture in Contemporary America*, Hanover, NH: Wesleyan University Press, 1994, 31.

15. Jacques Attali, *Noise: The Political Economy of Music*, 1977; English translation Minneapolis: University of Minnesota Press, 1985, 4.

16. Lois Stavsky, I. E. Mozeson, and Dani Reyes Mozeson, *The A 2 Z: The Book of Rap and Hip-Hop Slang*, New York: Boulevard Books, 1995, 72.
17. Ibid.
18. "Looking for the Perfect Beat," *The South Bank Show*, British ITV Series, broadcast in Los Angeles on the Bravo Cable Network, February 11, 1996. Transcription by Carolyn Cooper.
19. Geneva Smitherman, "'The Chain Remain the Same': Communicative Practices in the Hip Hop Nation," revised version of a paper presented at the English in Africa conference, Grahamstown Foundation, Monument Conference Center, Grahamstown, South Africa, September 11-14, 1995, 18-19.
20. The Fugees, "No Woman, No Cry," *The Score*, Columbia Records, 1996.
21. David Toop, *Rap Attack 2: African Rap to Global Hip Hop*, London: Serpent's Tale, 1991, 19.
22. Ibid., 18-19. On the significance of Harlem as African diasporic city par excellence, see, for example, the Jamaican Claude McKay's novel, *Home to Harlem*.
23. Dick Hebdige, *Cut 'N' Mix: Culture, Identity and Caribbean Music*, London: Routledge, 1987, 137.
24. Ibid.
25. Ibid., 138.
26. Ibid.
27. I am indebted to Louis Chude-Sokei for these examples.
28. "Pinkney" is inaccurate. The Jamaican word is "pikni."
29. I am indebted to Terri-Lynn Cross, former administrator, UCLA Center for African-American Studies, for informing me of these African American terms, which she speculates are of Portuguese origin.
30. Geneva Smitherman, *Black Talk: Words and Phrases from the Hood to the Amen Corner*, Boston: Houghton Mifflin, 1994, 51.
31. *The South Bank Show*, "Looking for the Perfect Beat," The British ITV Series, broadcast in Los Angeles on the Bravo Cable Network, Sunday, February 11, 1996. Transcription by Carolyn Cooper.
32. Buju Banton, *'Til Shiloh*, Loose Cannon/Polygram Records, 314-524 119-2, 1995
33. Frances Cress Welsing, *The Isis Papers: The Keys to the Colors*, Chicago: Third World Press, 1991, 110.
34. Cheryl L. Keyes, "'We're More than a Novelty, Boys': Strategies of Female Rappers in the Rap Music Tradition," in Joan Newlon Radner, ed., *Feminist Messages: Coding in Women's Folk Culture*, Urbana: University of Illinois Press, 1993, 216. Keyes quotes Roger Abrahams, "Negotiating Respect: Patterns of Presentation among Black Women," in Claire R. Farrer, ed. *Women and Folklore: Images and Genres*, Prospect Heights, IL: Waveland Press, 1975, 67.
35. "Looking for the Perfect Beat."

CHAPTER 9

1. Stuart Hall, "What Is This 'Black' in Black Popular Culture?" in David Morley and Kuan-Hsing Chen, eds., *Stuart Hall: Critical Dialogues in Cultural Studies*, London: Routledge, 1996, 469-70.

2. Apache Indian, "Don Raja," Track 1, *No Reservations*, Island Records, CID 8001 514 112-2, 1993. The transcription of the song texts given in the liner notes is not always accurate.

3. John Rex and Robert Moore, *Race, Community, and Conflict: A Study of Sparkbrook*, London: Oxford University Press, 1967, 19

4. Ibid., copyright page.

5. Ibid.

6. John Rex and Sally Tomlinson, *Colonial Immigrants in a British City: A Class Analysis*, London: Routledge & Kegan Paul, 1979, 72.

7. Ibid.

8. Ibid.

9. George Lipsitz, *Dangerous Crossroads: Popular Music, Postmodernism and the Poetics of Place*, London: Verso, 1994, 14-15.

10. Ibid., 15.

11. Michael Peter Smith, "Can You Imagine?: Transnational Migration and the Globalization of Grassroots Politics," *Social Text* 39 (Summer 1994): 15-16.

12. Ibid., 16.

13. *Gleaner*, April 19, 2001, C9.

14. Steel Pulse, "Roller Skates," Track 4, *Earth Crisis*, Elektra/Asylum, 9 60315-2, 1984.

15. In an unpublished paper, "Banking on Caribbean Talent: Intellectual Property Rights and the Entertainment Industry," Hubert Devonish and I examine the politics of appropriation in the music business. The paper was presented at the Business Conference of the Rotary Clubs of Jamaica and Port-of-Spain, held in Ocho Rios, Jamaica, in June 1995.

16. Louise Bennett, *Selected Poems*, ed. Mervyn Morris, Kingston: Sangster's, 1982; rpt 1983, 106.

17. Vivek Chaudhury, "Enter the Rajamuffins," *The Guardian*, September 19, 1995, 4. I am indebted to Cecil Gutzmore, former lecturer in Caribbean Studies at the University of North London, for research assistance for this chapter, locating primary texts.

18. Tony Thompson, "Yardies: Myth and Reality," *The Guardian*, September 19, 1995, 5.

19. Ibid.

20. Zadie Smith, *White Teeth*, London: Hamish Hamilton, 2000, 192.

21. Garry Mulholland, "Intriguing Outcastes," *The Guardian*, August 30, 1995, 8.

22. The orthography used in the liner notes is misleading; the spelling ought to be "bawl."

23. Problems of orthography, again; the spelling ought to be "cock." Apache Indian does pronounce the word in keeping with the "cork" spelling, but this is not accurate Jamaican.

24. Apache Indian, "Chok There," Track 2, *No Reservations*.

25. Apache Indian, "Come Follow Me," Track 8, *No Reservations*. The use of "man" here is somewhat ambiguous; it functions either to mark the gender of the "Indian man" or as the popular gender-neutral Jamaican interjection.

26. John R. Rickford, *Dimensions of a Creole Continuum: History, Texts & Linguistic Analysis of Guyanese Creole*, Stanford, CA: Stanford University Press, 1987, 65. I am indebted to Hubert Devonish for this reference.

27. Apache Indian, "Don Raja," Track 15, *No Reservations*. Again, the orthography used in the liner notes is misleading; the spelling ought to be "a." "Me are" is ungrammatical Jamaican.
28. Apache Indian, "Come Follow Me," Track 8, *No Reservations*.
29. Ibid.
30. Jerry Pinto, "No Reservations About Being an Indian: Apache Indian in Conversation with Jerry Pinto," *Illustrated Weekly of India*, June 12-18, 1993, 24.
31. Apache Indian, "Make Way for the Indian," Track 1, *Make Way for the Indian*, Mango, 162-539 948-2, 1995.
32. Pinto, "No Reservations About Being an Indian." Pinto seems to assume that Wild Apache Supercat is Native American. He is, in fact, Jamaican.
33. Apache Indian, "Badd Indian," Track 14, *No Reservations*.
34. Apache Waria with Arawak, "Mention," Track 9, *The Best of Apache Waria* Vol. 1, Waria Productions, AWCD-01, n.d.
35. Apache Indian, "Jump Up," Track 2, *Real People*, Warner Music Sweden, 3984 204562, 1997.
36. Apache Indian, "Mention," Track 7, *Real People*.
37. Apache Indian, "India (A.I.F.)," Track 8, *Real People*.
38. Ibid.
39. Ibid.
40. Pinto, "No Reservations About Being an Indian."
41. Apache Indian and Boy George, "In the Ghetto," Track 1, *Karma*, Sunset Records, SRCD011, 2000.
42. Ibid.
43. Apache Indian, "Religion," Track 3, *Karma*.
44. Apache Indian and Luciano, "Calling Out to Jah," Track 5, *Karma*.
45. Earl Lovelace, *The Dragon Can't Dance*, 1979; rpt London: Longman, 1983, 224.
46. Ibid.
47. Apache Indian, "Chok There," Track 2, No Reservations.

CHAPTER 10

1. Jean D'Costa and Barbara Lalla, eds., *Voices in Exile: Jamaican Texts of the 18th and 19th Centuries*, Tuscaloosa: University of Alabama Press, 1989, 6.
2. Quoted in ibid., 18.
3. Ibid., 132.
4. See quote below the English translation of Williams's Latin "Ode" to George Haldane, Esq.
5. Edward Long, *The History of Jamaica*, 1774; rpt. London: Frank Cass, 1970, Vol. 11, 476.
6. Quoted in D'Costa and Lalla, eds., *Voices in Exile*, 10-11.
7. Claude McKay, *My Green Hills of Jamaica*, Kingston: Heinemann, 1978, 66-7; cited in Winston James, *A Fierce Hatred of Injustice: Claude McKay's Jamaica and his Poetry of Rebellion*, Kingston: Ian Randle Publishers, 2001, 42-43.
8. Ibid.
9. Claude McKay, *Songs of Jamaica*: Gardner, 1912 and *Constab Ballads*, London: Watts, 1912.

10. Mary Jane Hewitt, "A Comparative Study of Zora Neale Hurston & Louise Bennett as Cultural Conservators," PhD. dissertation then in progress, University of the West Indies, Mona. Cited in Edward Kamau Brathwaite, *History of the Voice*, London: New Beacon Books, 1984, 28.
11. Louise Bennett, *Jamaica Labrish*, Kingston: Sangster's, 1966, 169.
12. Rex Nettleford, "Introduction," to Bennett, *Jamaica Labrish*, 9. For example, Professor the Hon. Rex Nettleford, in his 1966 introduction to Bennett's Jamaica Labrish, describes her experimental creative writing in Jamaican Creole thus – with a measure of irony one supposes: "In a quarter of a century she has carved designs out of the shapeless and unruly substance that is the Jamaican dialect." Nettleford, as a schoolboy at Cornwall College, carved dialect verse in the style of Louise Bennett.
13. Ibid., 10.
14. Ibid., 218-19.
15. Ibid.
16. Miss Lou, "Jamaica Language," Track 3, *"Yes M' Dear,"* Sonic Sounds Miami, SONCD-0079, n.d. This dramatic monologue is published in Louise Bennett, *Aunty Roachy Seh*, ed. Mervyn Morris, Kingston: Sangster's, 1993, 1-3.
17. Ibid., 1.
18. Ibid., 1-2.
19. Louise Bennett interviewed by Dennis Scott, "Bennett on Bennett," *Caribbean Quarterly* 14, 1-2 (1968): 98.
20. Frederic Cassidy, *Jamaica Talk*, London: Macmillan, 1961, 433.
21. Cassidy and LePage, *Dictionary of Jamaican English*, 1967, 1980, xxxvii-lxiv.
22. Mervyn Morris, "Printing the Performance," *Jamaica Journal* 23, 1 (1990): 22.
23. Carolyn Cooper, "Cho! Misa Cargill, Riispek Juu!" *Sunday Gleaner*, November 5, 1989, 8.
24. Authored by Carolyn Cooper.
25. Sean Reid, "Utter Rubbish, Dr. Cooper," *Jamaica Observer*, April 15, 1995, 8.
26. First presented at the Society for Caribbean Linguistics Conference, University of the West Indies, Mona, in August 2000; and in March 2002 at the European Association of Commonwealth Literature and Language Studies Conference, University of Copenhagen, to which I had been invited as a keynote speaker.
27. See, for example, Kathryn Brodber, "Dynamism and Assertiveness in the Public Voice: Turn-taking and Code-switching in Radio Talk Shows in Jamaica," *Pragmatics*, 2.4 (1992): 487-504.
28. Personal communication with Carolyn Cooper, 2003.
29. Statement made at a seminar on dub poetry, Jamaica School of Drama, January 17, 1986. Transcript of excerpts by Mervyn Morris.
30. Kamau Brathwaite, *History of the Voice*, London: New Beacon Books, 1984, 9.
31. Ibid., 13.
32. At the 1989 meeting of the U.K. Society for Caribbean Studies, where I presented an early version of the essay "Slackness Hiding from Culture: Erotic Play in the Dancehall," John Figueroa, editor of *Caribbean Voices* Vols. I & II, suggested that I publish the lyrics of the DJs in the sample. But given the limited readership of written texts in comparison to the wide audience for electronic recordings, it seemed to me at the time a retrograde step.
33. C. Renfrew, *Archaeology and Language: The Puzzle of Indo-European Languages*, London: Penguin Books, 1987, 182.

Works Cited

Adonijah. "Dub's Not the Force of All Evil," *Weekend Nation*, April 14, 2000, 13.

Attali, Jacques. *Noise: The Political Economy of Music*, 1977 (English translation), Minneapolis: University of Minnesota Press, 1985.

Bakere-Yusuf, Bibi. E-mail correspondence with author, January 10 and 13, 2003.

Banks, Ingrid. *Hair Matters: Beauty Power, and Black Consciousness*, New York: New York University Press, 2000.

Barbados Advocate Editorial. "Bottle Ban: Strict rules for Kensington," April 11, 2000, 1.

Barrow, Steve. *Tougher Than Tough: 35 Years of Jamaican Hits*, Island Records Box Set, 1993.

Baugh, Edward. *It Was the Singing*, Kingston: Sandberry Press, 2000.

Bennett, Louise. "Bennett on Bennett," interview with Dennis Scott, *Caribbean Quarterly* 14, 1-2 (1968): 97-101.

——. *Jamaica Labrish*, Kingston: Sangster's, 1966.

Best, Curwen. "Caribbean Music and the Discourse of AIDS," *Small Axe*, No. 3, March 1998, 57-63.

Boyne, Ian. "How Dancehall Promotes Violence," *Sunday Gleaner*, December 22, 2002, Section G1; G3.

——. "How Dancehall Holds Us Back," *Sunday Gleaner*, December 29, 2002, Section G 1; G5.

——. "'Bling-Bling Christianity Run Things," *Sunday Gleaner*, July 20, 2003, G2.

——. "True and Still Unspoilt Icon: The One and Only Miss Lou," *Sunday Gleaner*, August 3, 2003, G1; G3.

Brathwaite, Edward Kamau. *The Arrivants: A New World Trilogy*, Oxford: Oxford University Press, rpt. 1978.

——. *History of the Voice*, London: New Beacon Books, 1984.

Brodber, Kathryn. "Dynamism and Assertiveness in the Public Voice: Turn-taking and Code-switching in Radio Talk Shows in Jamaica," in *Pragmatics* 2, 4 (1992): 487-504.

Brown, Stewart, ed., *The Pressures of the Text: Orality, Texts and the Telling of Tales*, Birmingham: Centre of West African Studies, University of Birmingham, 1995.

Burton, Richard. *Afro-Creole: Power, Opposition and Play in the Caribbean*, Ithaca: Cornell University Press, 1997.

Carr, Robert. "On 'Judgements': Poverty, Sexuality-Based Violence and Human Rights in 21st Century Jamaica," *The Caribbean Journal of Social Work* 2 (July 2003): 71-87.

Cassidy, Frederic. *Jamaica Talk,* Institute of Jamaica/Macmillan, 1961.

Chaudhury, Vivek. "Enter the Rajamuffins," *The Guardian,* September 19, 1995, 4.

Clunis, Andrew. "Banned: London pressures dancehall stars." *The Sunday Gleaner.* June 27, 2004. A1.

Conally, Michael. "Defen' it." *Pure Class (Jamaica Herald's* Sunday magazine), November 29, 1992, 12.

Constable, Catherine. "Making Up the Truth: On Lies, Lipstick and Friedrich Nietzsche," in Stella Bruzzi and Pamela Church Gibson, eds., *Fashion Cultures: Theories, Explorations and Analysis,* London: Routledge, 2000, 191-200.

Cooke, Melville. "Ninja Man, Reneto Adams—Both above the Law." *Gleaner,* January 3, 2003, A4.

Cooper, Carolyn. "Peter Tosh Interview," *Pulse* (June 1984): 12; 14; 15; 32.

————. "Cho! Misa Cargill, Riispek Juu!," *Sunday Gleaner,* November 5, 1989, 8.

————. "War on Ignorance," *Sunday Advocate,* April 16, 2001, 13.

————. *Noises in the Blood: Orality, Gender and the "Vulgar" Body of Jamaican Popular Culture,* London: Macmillan, 1993; 1994; Durham: Duke University Press, 1995, 2000.

————. "Race and the Cultural Politics of Self-Representation: A View from the University of the West Indies," *Research in African Literatures,* 27, 4 (1996): 97-105.

Cooper, Carolyn and Hubert Devonish. "Banking on Caribbean Talent: Intellectual Property Rights and the Entertainment Industry," unpublished paper presented at the Business Conference of the Rotary Clubs of Jamaica and Port-of-Spain, Ocho Rios, Jamaica, June 1995.

Cooper, Wayne F., ed. *The Passion of Claude McKay: Selected Poetry and Prose, 1912-1948,* New York: Schocken Books, 1973.

Cowell, Julian. "Jamaicans in U.S. Prisons," *Abeng Newsletter* 3, 1 (January-March 1998): 10.

Cruden, Alexander. *Complete Concordance to the Old and New Testament,* London: Frederick Warne, 3rd edition, 1769, 166.

Cummings, Mark, "I have learnt my lesson—Sean Paul," *Daily Observer,* August 13, 2003, 25.

Daily Observer, "Children's homes review ordered: Study to determine if Ja meeting UN child rights obligations, " December 31, 2002, 1.

Davidson, Vernon. "Charles Offers Solution to Street Vending Problem," *Daily Observer,* January 1, 2003, 3.

Davis, Stephen. *Reggae Bloodlines: In Search of the Music and Culture of Jamaica,* 1977; London: Heinemann Educational Books, rpt. 1981.

D'Costa, Jean and Barbara Lalla, eds. *Voices in Exile: Jamaican Texts of the 18th and 19th Centuries*, Tuscaloosa: University of Alabama Press, 1989.

Editorial, "Bad Product: Don't Import the Garbage," *Barbados Advocate*, April 10, 2000, 8.

Editorial, "Vile Vocals: Unofficial War in Bim," *Barbados Advocate*, April 11, 2000, 8.

Emecheta, Buchi. *The Joys of Motherhood*, 1979; London: Heinemann, rpt. 1980.

Fanon, Frantz. *Black Skin, White Masks*, 1952; New York: Grove Press, rpt. 1967.

Fineman, Mark. "Attack Points to 'Lethal' Mix of Religion, Rebellion, Drugs." *Los Angeles Times*, January 7, 2001, 1A.

Frederic, Cassidy and Robert LePage, *Dictionary of Jamaican English*, Cambridge: Cambridge University Press, 1967; 1980.

"Free Thinker" (letter to the editor). "Right to hold an opinion," *Gleaner*, March 8, 1993, 7.

Gleaner, April 19, 2001, photo, C9.

Green, Cordell. E-mail correspondence with author, June 11, 2003.

Gutzmore, Cecil. "'Incline Thine Ear': Roots, Reality and Culture in Jamaican Dancehall DJ Music," Bob Marley Lecture, University of the West Indies, Mona, Jamaica, unpublished, February 2002.

Hall, Stuart. "What is this 'Black' in Black Popular Culture?" in David Morley and Kuan-Hsing Chen, eds., *Stuart Hall: Critical Dialogues in Cultural Studies*, London: Routledge, 1996, 465-475.

———. "Cultural Studies and the Politics of Internationalization," an interview with Kuan-Hsing Chen, in David Morley and Kuan-Hsing Chen, eds., *Stuart Hall: Critical Dialogues in Cultural Studies*, London: Routledge, 1996, 392-408.

Hebdige, Dick. *Cut 'N' Mix: Culture, Identity and Caribbean Music*, London: Routledge, 1987.

Henry, Balford. "Bob and Bounty," *Weekend Star*, February 5, 1999, 23.

Henry, William. "Reggae/Dancehall Music as an autonomous space for cultural expression," BA Dissertation, Goldsmiths College, London University, 1997.

Hogg, Donald. "The Convince Cult in Jamaica," *Yale University Publications in Anthropology* 58, 3-24. Reprinted in Sidney Mintz, comp., *Papers in Caribbean Anthropology*, New Haven: Human Relations Area Files Press, 1970.

Hope, Donna. "Inna Di Dancehall Dis/place: Socio-Cultural Politics of Identity in Jamaica," Masters of Philosophy Thesis, University of the West Indies, Mona, 2001.

Humm, Maggie. "Is the Gaze Feminist? Pornography, Film and Feminism" in Gary Day and Clive Bloom, eds., *Perspectives on Pornography: Sexuality in Film and Literature*, London: Macmillan, 1988, 69-82.

James, Winston and Clive Harris eds., *Inside Babylon: The Caribbean Diaspora in Britain*, London: Verso, 1993.

James, Winston. *A Fierce Hatred of Injustice: Claude McKay's Jamaica and his Poetry of Rebellion*, Kingston: Ian Randle Publishers, 2001.

Jekyll, Walter ed. *Jamaican Song and Story*, London: David Nutt, 1907.

Johnson, Linton Kwesi. "Introduction" to *Tougher Than Tough: The Story of Jamaican Music,* Island Records Box Set, 1993, 5.

Keyes, Cheryl L. "'We're More than a Novelty, Boys': Strategies of Female Rappers in the Rap Music Tradition," in Joan Newlon Radner, ed. *Feminist Messages: Coding in Women's Folk Culture,* Urbana and Chicago: University of Illinois Press, 1993.

Kincaid, Jamaica. *Annie John,* New York: Farrar, Straus and Giroux, 1983.

———. *Lucy,* New York: Farrar, Straus and Giroux, 1990.

Lake, Obiagele. *Rastafari Women: Subordination in the Midst of Liberation Theology,* Durham: Carolina Academic Press, 1998.

Lalla, Barbara. *Defining Jamaican Fiction: Marronage and the Discourse of Survival,* Tuscaloosa: The University of Alabama Press, 1996.

Lamming, George. *In the Castle of My Skin,* London: Longman, Caribbean, 1992; reprint of Michael Joseph, 1953.

Lipsitz, George. *Dangerous Crossroads: Popular Music, Postmodernism and the Poetics of Place,* London: Verso, 1994.

Long, Edward. *The History of Jamaica,* 1774; London: Frank Cass, rpt. 1970, Vol. II.

Lovelace, Earl. *The Dragon Can't Dance,* 1979; London: Longman, rpt. 1985.

Mackey, Nathaniel. "An Interview with Kamau Brathwaite" in Stewart Brown, ed., *The Art of Kamau Brathwaite,* Mid Glamorgan: Seren, 1995, 13-32.

Mandingo. "The Origins and Meanings of Dancehall & Ragamuffin," *Dance Hall,* February 1994, 14.

Mapp, Ben. "First Reggae. Then Rap. Now it's Dancehall," *New York Times,* June 21, 1992, 24-28.

McKay, Claude. *Home to Harlem,* 1928; Chatham, New Jersey: The Chatham Bookseller, rpt. 1973.

Meschino, Patricia. "The Marley Brothers Shining Sons," *Rhythm Magazine,* Issue 86 (June 2000): 27.

Morris, Mervyn. "Printing the Performance," *Jamaica Journal* 23.1 (1990) : 21-26.

———, ed., Louise Bennett, *Selected Poems,* Kingston: Sangster's, 1982; rpt 1983.

———, ed., Louise Bennett, *Aunty Roachy Seh,* Kingston: Sangster's, 1993.

Mulholland, Garry. "Intriguing Outcastes," *The Guardian,* August 30, 1995, 8.

Myrie, Iris. "Distasteful side of dancehall music," *Gleaner,* February 14, 2003, A5.

Nelson, Cary, Paula A. Treichler, and Lawrence Grossberg, eds. *Cultural Studies,* New York: Routledge, 1992.

Nettleford, Rex. "Introduction" to Louise Bennett, *Jamaica Labrish,* Kingston: Sangster's, 1966, 9-24.

———. "War, Recession and Gorillas (Tourism Madness Indeed!)," *Gleaner,* January 16, 1991, 19B.

Noble, Denise. "Ragga Music: Dis/Respecting Black Women and Dis/Reputable Sexualities," in Barnor Hesse, ed., *Un/settled Multiculturalisms: Diasporas, Entanglements, Transruptions,* London: Zed Books, 2000, 148-169.

Noel, Peter. "Batty Boys in Babylon," *Village Voice* xxxviii, 2 (January 12, 1993): 36.

Oyewumi, Oyeronke. *The Invention of Women: Making an African Sense of Western Gender Discourses,* Minneapolis: University of Minnesota Press, 1997.

Papa Pilgrim. "Reggae Sunsplash 93: Report From Yard," *The Beat* 12, 5 (1993): 46-50.

Pierson, Ransdell. "'Kill Gays' Hit Song Stirs Fury," *New York Post,* October 24-October 25, 1992, 5.

Pinto, Jerry. "No Reservations About Being an Indian: Apache Indian in Conversation with Jerry Pinto," *Illustrated Weekly of India,* June 12-18, 1993, 24-25.

Reid, Sean. "Utter Rubbish, Dr. Cooper," *Jamaica Observer,* April 15, 1995, 8.

Renfrew, C., *Archaeology and Language: The Puzzle of Indo-European Languages,* London: Penguin Books, 1987.

Rex, John and Robert Moore, *Race, Community, and Conflict: A Study of Sparkbrook,* London: Oxford University Press, 1967.

Rex, John and Sally Tomlinson, *Colonial Immigrants in a British City: A Class Analysis,* London: Routledge & Kegan Paul, 1979.

Rickford, John R. *Dimensions of a Creole Continuum: History, Texts & Linguistic Analysis of Guyanese Creole.* Stanford: Stanford University Press, 1987.

Ritch, Dawn. "Tourism Madness," *Sunday Gleaner,* January 13, 1991, 8A.

Rivera, Raquel. *New York Ricans from the Hip Hop Zone,* New York: Palgrave Macmillan, 2003.

Rohlehr, Gordon. "Bridges of Sound: An Approach to Edward Brathwaite's 'Jah'," *Caribbean Quarterly* 26, 1-2 (1980), 13-31.

———. "Folk Research: Fossil or Living Bone?" *Massachusetts Review,* Autumn-Winter 1994, 383-395.

Rose, Tricia. *Black Noise: Rap Music and Black Culture in Contemporary America,* Hanover, N.H.: Wesleyan University Press, 1994.

Ross, Andrew. *Real Love: In Pursuit of Cultural Justice,* New York: New York University Press, 1998.

Scott, David. "'Wi a di Govament': An Interview with Anthony B," *Small Axe* 2 (September 1997): 79-101.

Senior, Olive. *Arrival of the Snake-Woman and Other Stories,* London: Longman Caribbean, 1989.

Smith, Michael Peter. "Can You Imagine?: Transnational Migration and the Globalization of Grassroots Politics," *Social Text* 39 (Summer 1994).

Smith, Zadie. *White Teeth,* London: Hamish Hamilton, 2000.

Smitherman, Geneva. *Black Talk: Words and Phrases from the Hood to the Amen Corner,* Houghton Mifflin, 1994.

Smitherman, Geneva. "'The Chain Remain the Same': Communicative Practices in the Hip Hop Nation." Revised version of an unpublished paper presented at the English in Africa Conference, Grahamstown Foundation, Monument Conference Center, Grahamstown, South Africa, September 11-14, 1995.

The South Bank Show, "Looking for the Perfect Beat," The British ITV Series, broadcast in Los Angeles on the Bravo Cable Network, Sunday, February 11, 1996. Transcription by Carolyn Cooper.

Stallybrass, Peter and Allon White. *The Politics and Poetics of Transgression*, Ithaca, New York: Cornell University Press, 1986.

Stavsky, Lois, I.E. Mozeson, and Dani Reyes Mozeson. *The A 2 Z: The Book of Rap and Hip-Hop Slang*, New York: Boulevard Books, 1995.

Stolzoff, Norman. *Wake the Town and Tell the People: Dancehall Culture in Jamaica*, Durham: Duke University Press, 2000.

Tate, Greg. *Flyboy in the Buttermilk: Essays on Contemporary America*, New York: Fireside Simon & Schuster, 1992.

Teish, Luisah. *Carnival of the Spirit*, San Francisco: Harper, 1994.

Thelwell, Michael. *The Harder They Come*, London: Pluto, 1980.

Thompson, Tony. "Yardies: Myth and Reality," *The Guardian*, September 19, 1995, 5.

Toop, David. *Rap Attack 2: African Rap to Global Hip Hop*, London: Serpent's Tale, 1991.

Warner-Lewis, Maureen. *Central Africa in the Caribbean: Transcending Time, Transforming Cultures*. Kingston, Jamaica: University of the West Indies Press, 2003.

Watts, Corneldi. "Ban the nasty lyrics," *Barbados Advocate*, June 23, 2002, 11.

Weekend Observer, "'Shiprider' takes effect Tuesday," March 6, 1998, 4.

Wesling, Frances Cress. *The Isis Papers: The Keys to the Colors*, Chicago: Third World Press, 1991.

West, Cornel. *Race Matters*, Boston: Beacon Press, 1993.

White, Garth. "Traditional Musical Practice in Jamaica and its Influence on the Birth of Modern Jamaican Popular Music," African-Caribbean Institute of Jamaica monograph; extracted from *ACIJ Newsletter* 7 (March 1982).

Willis, Tom. "From Ragga to Riches," *Sunday Times* (London) April 4, 1993.

Zabihyan, Kimi. "A roar from the lion's den," interview with Buju Banton, *The Guardian*, Friday Review, December 8, 1995, 14.

DISCOGRAPHY

Alexander, Monty. "Cowboys Talk," Track 5, *Caribbean Circle*, Chesky Records, JD80, 1992.

Anthony B. *Real Revolutionary*, Greensleeves, GRELCD 230, 1996; apparently issued as *So Many Things* by VP in the United States.

———. *Universal Struggle*, VP Records, VPCD 1510 2, 1997.

Apache Indian. *No Reservations,* Island Records, 1993.

———. *Make Way for the Indian,* Mango, 162-539 948-2, 1995.

———. *Real People,* Warner Music Sweden, 3984 204562, 1997.

———. *Karma,* Sunset Records, SRCD011, 2000.

Apache Waria with Arawak. "Mention," Track 9, *The Best of Apache Waria,* Vol. 1, Waria Productions, AWCD-01, n.d.

Beenie Man. *Blessed,* Island Records, IJCD 3005/524 138-2, 1995.

Bennett, Louise. Miss Lou. "Jamaica Language," Track 3, *"Yes M' Dear,"* Sonic Sounds Miami, SONCD-0079, n.d.

Bounty Killer. *Ghetto Dictionary: The Mystery,* VP Records, VPCD 1681, 2002.

Buju Banton, "Boom Bye Bye," Track 1, *Strictly the Best,* Vol. 9, VP Records, VPCD 1291, 1993.

Buju Banton. *Voice of Jamaica,* Mercury, 518 013-2, 1993.

———. *Mr Mention,* Polygram Records, 522 022 – 2, 1994.

———. *'Til Shiloh,* Loose Cannon/Polygram Records, 314-524 119-2, 1995

———. "I.C.I.," Track 4, *Cell Block,* Vol. 2, Penthouse Records, CBCD2032, 1995.

———. *Friends for Life,* VP Records/Atlantic, 0 7567 83634 2, 2003.

———. "Gal You Body Good," Track 1, *Buju Banton Meets Garnett Silk and Tony Rebel at the Super Stars Conference,* Rhino Records, RNCD 2033 n.d.

Capleton. *One Mission,* J & D Distributors, JDCD 0013, 1999.

———. *More Fire,* VP Records, VPCD 1587, 2000.

Ce'Cile. "Do It To Me," King of Kings label, 2003.

Cocoa Tea. "No Threat," Track 6, *Little Sound Boy,* VP Records, VPCD 1441, 1996.

Gonzalez, Fernando. Liner notes to Danilo Perez, *Central Avenue,* Impulse, IMCD 279, 1998.

Hammond, Beres. *Music is Life,* VP Records, VPCD1624, 2001.

Lady Saw. *Give Me the Reason,* Diamond Rush, RUSHCD1, 1996.

Marley, Bob. *Burnin',* Tuff Gong Records, 422-846 200-2, 1973.

———. *Catch a Fire,* Tuff Gong Records, 422-846 201-2, 1973.

———. *Natty Dread,* Tuff Gong Records, 422-846 204-2, 1974.

———. *Rastaman Vibration,* Tuff Gong Records, 422-846 205-2, 1976.

———. *Exodus,* Tuff Gong Records, 422-846 208-2, 1977.

———. *Survival,* Tuff Gong Records, 422-846 202-2, 1979.

———. *Uprising,* Tuff Gong Records, 422-846 211-2, 1980.

———. Interview with Dermott Hussey, Track 20, *Talkin' Blues,* Tuff Gong Records, 422-848 243-2, 1991.

Niney. "Blood and Fire," Track 15, *Reggae Hit the Town,* CD 2, *Tougher than Tough : The Story of Jamaican Music,* Island Records, CD2 518 401-2, 1993.

Ninjaman. *Warning You Now*, Jammy$ Records, 1990.

———. "Test the High Power," Track 2, *Little Sound Boy*, VP Records, VPCD1441, 1996.

Pan Head and Sugar Black. "A Wi Run the Gun Them," Track 20, *Buju Banton Meets Garnett Silk and Tony Rebel at the Super Stars Conference*, Rhino Records, RNCD 2033, n.d.

Prezident Brown and Don Yute, "African Ting," Track 10, *Prezident Selections*, RUNNetherlands, RNN0043, n.d.

Shabba Ranks. *As Raw as Ever*, Sony, 468102 2, 1991.

———. *Just Reality*, Vine Yard Records, VYDCD 6, 1991.

———. *Rough & Ready, Vol. 1*, Sony 471442 2, 1992.

———. *X-Tra Naked*, Sony, EK 52464, 1992.

Spragga Benz and Elephant Man. "Warrior Cause," Track 6, *Strictly The Best*, Vol. 27, VP Records, VPCD1639, 2001.

Steel Pulse. "Roller Skates," Track 4, *Earth Crisis*, Elektra/Asylum, 9 60315-2, 1984.

Sugar Minott. "Can't Cross The Border," Track 7, *Little Sound Boy*, VP Records, VPCD 1441, 1996.

Terror Fabulous. "Praise Jah & Live," Track 2, *Kette Drum*, Digital B, DBCD 2039, n.d.

TOK, "Chi-Chi Man," Track 4, *Reggae Gold 2001*, VP Records, VPCD 1629, 2001.

The Ethiopians, "Gun Man," Track 12, *The Ethiopians*, Trojan Records, CDTRL 228,1988; 1986.

The Fugees. *The Score*, Columbia Records, 1996.

Tony Rebel. "Chatty Chatty," Track 9, *Just Ragga*, Charm Records, CRCD14, 1992.

Tosh, Peter. "Equal Rights," Track 5, *Equal Rights*, CBS Records, CK 34670, 1977

VIDEOGRAPHY

Babymother, Dir. Julian Henriques, Formation Films, Film Four Distributors, 1998.

Dancehall Queen, Dirs. Rick Elgood and Don Letts, Island Jamaica Films, Island Digital Media, 1997.

The Darker Side of Black, Dir. Isaac Julien, Black Audio Film Collective, 1994.

Lee, Sandra, Interviewed by Anthony Miller, "Entertainment Report," Television Jamaica, broadcast on April 23, 1999.

Life and Debt, Dir. Stephanie Black, Tuff Gong Pictures, 2001.

One Love, Dirs. Rick Elgood and Don Letts, UK Film Council, 2003.

Third World Cop, Dir. Christopher Browne, Palm Pictures, 1999.

Permissions

Ltd. and by Fairwood Music, Ltd. (PRS) for the rest of the world on behalf of Blue
Mountain Music, Ltd.

Pimper's Paradise

(Bob Marley)

© 1980 Fifty Six Hope Road / Odnil Music Limited (ASCAP). All rights for North America
controlled by Fairwood Music USA (ASCAP) on behalf of Blue Mountain Music,
Ltd. and by Fairwood Music, Ltd. (PRS) for the rest of the world on behalf of Blue
Mountain Music, Ltd.

Kinky Reggae

(Bob Marley)

© 1975 Fifty Six Hope Road / Odnil Music Limited (ASCAP). All rights for North America
controlled by Fairwood Music USA (ASCAP) on behalf of Blue Mountain Music,
Ltd. and by Fairwood Music, Ltd. (PRS) for the rest of the world on behalf of Blue
Mountain Music, Ltd.

Burnin' and Lootin'

(Bob Marley)

© 1974 Fifty Six Hope Road / Odnil Music Limited (ASCAP). All rights for North America
controlled by Fairwood Music USA (ASCAP) on behalf of Blue Mountain Music,
Ltd. and by Fairwood Music, Ltd. (PRS) for the rest of the world on behalf of Blue
Mountain Music, Ltd.

Ride Natty Ride

(Bob Marley)

© 1979 Fifty Six Hope Road / Odnil Music Limited (ASCAP). All rights for North America
controlled by Fairwood Music USA (ASCAP) on behalf of Blue Mountain Music,
Ltd. and by Fairwood Music, Ltd. (PRS) for the rest of the world on behalf of Blue
Mountain Music, Ltd.

One Love

(Bob Marley)

© 1968 Fifty Six Hope Road / Odnil Music Limited (ASCAP). All rights for North America
controlled by Fairwood Music USA (ASCAP) on behalf of Blue Mountain Music,
Ltd. and by Fairwood Music, Ltd. (PRS) for the rest of the world on behalf of Blue
Mountain Music, Ltd.

Who The Cap Fit

(Aston Barrett / Carleton Barrett)

© 1976 Fifty Six Hope Road / Odnil Music Limited (ASCAP). All rights for North America
controlled by Fairwood Music USA (ASCAP) on behalf of Blue Mountain Music,
Ltd. and by Fairwood Music, Ltd. (PRS) for the rest of the world on behalf of Blue
Mountain Music, Ltd.

War

(Aston Barrett / Carleton Barrett)

The photo of Apache Indian in Chapter 9 was taken by Joseph Chielli for Church Street Studios—Philadelphia, PA. Copyright sunset entertainment group 2003 / www.karmasound.com.

The photos listed below appear courtesy of Gleaner Co. Ltd., Kingston, Jamaica.

The photo appearing in the Introduction was taken by Dennis Coke.

The photos appearing in Chapters 1 and 8 were taken by Carlington Wilmot.

The photos appearing in Chapters 2, 5, and 7 were taken by Ian Allen.

The photo appearing in Chapter 3 was taken by Rudolph Brown.

The photo appearing in Chapter 4 was taken by Winston Sill.

The photographers for the photographs in chapters 6 and 10 are unknown.

The unpublished Ras Dizzy letters appear courtesy of Ras Dizzy.

Index